Complications in Dentoalveolar Surgery

Guest Editors

DENNIS-DUKE R. YAMASHITA, DDS
JAMES P. MCANDREWS, DDS

ORAL AND MAXILLOFACIAL SURGERY
CLINICS OF NORTH AMERICA

www.oralmaxsurgery.theclinics.com

Consulting Editor
RICHARD H. HAUG, DDS

August 2011 • Volume 23 • Number 3

SAUNDERS an imprint of ELSEVIER, Inc.

W.B. SAUNDERS COMPANY
A Division of Elsevier Inc.

1600 John F. Kennedy Blvd. • Suite 1800 • Philadelphia, PA 19103-2899

www.oralmaxsurgery.theclinics.com

ORAL AND MAXILLOFACIAL SURGERY CLINICS OF NORTH AMERICA Volume 23, Number 3
August 2011 ISSN 1042-3699, ISBN-13: 978-1-4557-1043-0

Editor: John Vassallo; j.vassallo@elsevier.com
Developmental Editor: Teia Stone

Oral and Maxillofacial Surgery Clinics of North America (ISSN 1042-3699) is published quarterly by Elsevier Inc., 360 Park Avenue South, New York, NY 10010-1710. Months of issue are February, May, August, and November. Business and Editorial Offices: 1600 John F. Kennedy Blvd., Suite 1800, Philadelphia, PA 19103-2899. Periodicals postage paid at New York, NY and additional mailing offices. Subscription prices are $329.00 per year for US individuals, $490.00 per year for US institutions, $147.00 per year for US students and residents, $383.00 per year for Canadian individuals, $583.00 per year for Canadian institutions, $441.00 per year for international individuals, $583.00 per year for international institutions and $200.00 per year for Canadian and foreign students/residents. To receive student/resident rate, orders must be accompanied by name or affiliated institution, date of term, and the *signature* of program/residency coordinator on institution letterhead. Orders will be billed at individual rate until proof of status is received. Foreign air speed delivery is included in all *Clinics* subscription prices. All prices are subject to change without notice. **POSTMASTER:** Send address changes to *Oral and Maxillofacial Surgery Clinics of North America,* Elsevier Periodicals Customer Service, 11830 Westline Industrial Drive, St. Louis, MO 63146. Tel: 1-800-654-2452 (U.S. and Canada); 314-447-8871 (outside U.S. and Canada). Fax: 314-447-8029. E-mail: journalscustomerservice-usa@elsevier.com (for print support); journalsonlinesupport-usa@elsevier.com (for online support).

Reprints. For copies of 100 or more, of articles in this publication, please contact the Commercial Reprints Department, Elsevier Inc., 360 Park Avenue South, New York, NY 10010-1710. Tel.: 212-633-3812; Fax: 212-462-1935; Email: reprints@elsevier.com.

Oral and Maxillofacial Surgery Clinics of North America is covered in MEDLINE/PubMed (*Index Medicus*).

Printed and bound by CPI Group (UK) Ltd, Croydon, CR0 4YY

Transferred to Digital Print 2011

Contributors

CONSULTING EDITOR

RICHARD H. HAUG, DDS
Carolinas Center for Oral Health, Charlotte,
North Carolina

GUEST EDITORS

**DENNIS-DUKE R. YAMASHITA, DDS,
FACD, FICD**
Professor of Dentistry; Director, Advanced
Program in Oral and Maxillofacial Surgery,
Division of Endodontics, Orthodontics and
Maxillofacial Surgery, Herman Ostrow School
of Dentistry of University of Southern California
and Los Angeles County/University of
Southern California Medical Center;
Co-Director of Dentistry, Los Angeles County/
University of Southern California Medical
Center; Section Chair, University of Southern
California University Hospital, Los Angeles,
California

**JAMES P. MCANDREWS, DDS,
FACD, FICD**
Assistant Clinical Professor, Oral and
Maxillofacial Surgery, Division of
Endodontics, Orthodontics and Maxillofacial
Surgery, Herman Ostrow School of Dentistry
of University of Southern California and
Los Angeles County/University of Southern
California Medical Center, Los Angeles,
California

AUTHORS

GERALD ALEXANDER, DDS
Attending Surgeon, Private Practice;
Department of Oral and Maxillofacial Surgery,
University of California, San Francisco; Oral
Maxillofacial Surgery Consultant, Veterans
Affairs Medical Center Fresno, Fresno, California

LEON A. ASSAEL, DMD
Professor and Chairman; Residency
Program Director, Oral and Maxillofacial
Surgery; Professor of Surgery, School of
Medicine; Medical Director, Hospital
Dentistry, Oregon Health and Science
University, Portland, Oregon

HANY ATTIA, DDS
Chief Resident, Department of Oral and
Maxillofacial Surgery, University of
California, San Francisco, California

THOMAS G. AUYONG, DDS
Clinical Assistant Professor, Department
of Hospital Affairs, Herman Ostrow School
of Dentistry, University of Southern California,
Los Angeles, California

JOSEPH BRUNWORTH, MD
Department of Otolaryngology–Head and
Neck Surgery, University of California
Irvine School of Medicine, Orange,
California

DAVID R. CUMMINGS, DDS, FACD
Assistant Clinical Professor, Department
of Oral and Maxillofacial Surgery,
University of Southern California
School of Dentistry, Los Angeles County/
University of Southern California Medical
Center; Private Practice, Mission Viejo,
California

ARTHUR W. CURLEY, JD
Assistant Professor, Dental Jurisprudence,
Arthur A. Dugoni School of Dentistry, University
of the Pacific, San Francisco; President and
Senior Trial Counsel, Bradley, Curley, Asiano,
Barrabee, Abel & Kowalski, P.C., Larkspur,
California

JEFFREY S. DEAN, DDS, MD, FACS
Program Director, Department of Oral and
Maxillofacial Surgery, Loma Linda University,
Loma Linda, California

JEFFREY HAMMOUDEH, MD, DDS
Assistant Professor, Division of Plastic and
Maxillofacial Surgery, Department of
Surgery, Children's Hospital Los Angeles,
Keck School of Medicine, University
of Southern California, Los Angeles,
California

ALAN S. HERFORD, DDS, MD, FACS
Chairman, Department of Oral and
Maxillofacial Surgery, Loma Linda University,
Loma Linda, California

PETER A. KRAKOWIAK, DMD, FRCD(C)
Clinical Assistant Professor, Oral and
Maxillofacial Surgery, Herman Ostrow
School of Dentistry, University of Southern
California, Los Angeles; Private Practice,
Lake Elsinore; Private Practice, Bonsall,
California

ANH LE, DDS, PhD
Associate Professor, Departments of
Oral and Maxillofacial Surgery; Center
for Craniofacial Molecular Biology,
Herman Ostrow School of Dentistry of the
University of Southern California,
Los Angeles, California

MICHAEL LYPKA, MD, DMD
Assistant Professor, Division of Pediatric
Plastic and Craniofacial Surgery, Department
of Pediatric Surgery; Division of Plastic and
Reconstructive Surgery, Department of
Surgery, University of Texas Medical School
at Houston, Houston, Texas

JAY P. MALMQUIST, DMD, FACD, FICD
Private Practice, Portland, Oregon

**JAMES P. MCANDREWS, DDS,
FACD, FICD**
Assistant Clinical Professor, Oral and
Maxillofacial Surgery, Division of
Endodontics, Orthodontics and Maxillofacial
Surgery, Herman Ostrow School of Dentistry
of University of Southern California and
Los Angeles County/University of Southern
California Medical Center, Los Angeles,
California

RAYMOND J. MELROSE, DDS
Emeritus Professor of Pathology, University
of Southern California; President and
Co-Owner, Oral Pathology Associates, Inc.,
Los Angeles, California

KARLA O'DELL, MD
Department of Otolaryngology–Head and
Neck Surgery, University of Southern
California, Los Angeles, California

TERRY Y. SHIBUYA, MD, FACS
Department of Otolaryngology–Head and
Neck Surgery, University of California
Irvine School of Medicine, Orange;
Department of Head and Neck Surgery,
Southern California Permanente Medical
Group, Anaheim, California

UTTAM SINHA, MD, FACS
Program Director, Department of
Otolaryngology–Head and Neck Surgery,
University of Southern California,
Los Angeles, California

**DENNIS-DUKE R. YAMASHITA,
DDS, FACD, FICD**
Professor of Dentistry; Director, Advanced
Program in Oral and Maxillofacial Surgery,
Division of Endodontics, Orthodontics and
Maxillofacial Surgery, Herman Ostrow
School of Dentistry of University of Southern
California and Los Angeles County/University
of Southern California Medical Center;
Co-Director of Dentistry, Los Angeles County/
University of Southern California Medical
Center; Section Chair, University of Southern
California University Hospital, Los Angeles,
California

Contents

> Local anesthetics are used routinely in oral and maxillofacial surgery. Local anesthetics are safe and effective drugs but do have risks that practitioners need to be aware of. This article reviews the complications of local anesthesia. A brief history is provided and the regional and systemic complications that can arise from using local anesthesia are discussed. These complications include paresthesia, ocular complications, allergies, toxicity, and methemoglobinemia. Understanding the risks involved with local anesthesia decreases the chances of adverse events occurring and ultimately leads to improved patient care.

> Displaced objects can occur in the practice of almost all procedures performed in the scope of oral and maxillofacial surgery. Anticipation of such occurrences is the hallmark of their prevention. The institution of proper techniques can help in reducing such occurrences. Knowledge of the techniques available in treating these incidences can greatly assist in their resolutions. This article sheds light on the prevention and management of such dreaded mishaps.

> Oral and maxillofacial surgeons perform a wide variety of surgical procedures. One of the major complications of these various surgical techniques is uncontrolled bleeding. The best management of perioperative hemorrhage is prevention. This includes proper preoperative patient evaluation, knowledge of the various bleeding disorders, and the characterization of the correct methods of management. This article evaluates various causes of bleeding, and identifies both local and systemic and pathways. Considerations of treatment for patients with these various disorders are discussed regarding the best management options for adequate hemostasis.

> Nerve injury associated with dentoalveolar surgery is a complication contributing to the altered sensation of the lower lip, chin, buccal gingivae, and tongue. This surgery-related sensory defect is a morbid postoperative outcome. Several risk factors have been proposed. This article reviews the incidence of trigeminal nerve injury, presurgical risk assessment, classification, and surgical coronectomy versus conventional extraction as an approach to prevent neurosensory damage associated with dentoalveolar surgery.

use, and the assessment of osteonecrosis incidence, pathophysiology, with some insights into treatment.

Osteoradionecrosis (ORN) is a severe complication of radiation therapy for head and neck cancer. The current theory in its pathophysiology is thought to be radiation-induced fibroatrophy of the bone. Location of primary tumor, stage of cancer, dose of radiation, oral hygiene, and smoking and alcohol use are risk factors in the development of ORN. Prevention is focused on thorough dental care before, during, and after radiation therapy. Treatment ranges from conservative management with oral rinses and local debridement to radical resection with microvascular free tissue transfer and reconstruction.

The routine submission of abnormal tissue for histopathologic diagnosis is a vital link in the appropriate management of patients. Receipt of a biopsy report brings the usual case to its full conclusion. Patients are best served when clinical impressions are verified by histopathologic examination, and this in turn will reduce the likelihood of successful malpractice litigation for failure or delay in diagnosis.

Complications are an inherent part of oral and maxillofacial surgery. A risk in surgery is a complication that occurs despite treatment that meets or exceeds the professional standard of care. When treatment fails to meet the standard of care, a complication may be considered the result of malpractice, resulting in claims for compensation. Whether a surgical procedure meets the standard of care is determined by expert witnesses evaluating the evidence. This article reviews legal issues and cases where complications have resulted in claims of malpractice. Recommendations for patient communication and documentation to reduce or eliminate such claims are presented.

Oral and Maxillofacial Surgery Clinics of North America

FORTHCOMING ISSUES

November 2011

Unanswered Questions in Oral and Maxillofacial Infections
Thomas R. Flynn, DMD,
Guest Editor

February 2012

Rhinoplasty: Current Therapy
Shahrokh C. Bagheri, DMD, MD, FACS,
Husain Ali Khan, DMD, MD and
Angelo Cuzalina, MD, *Guest Editors*

May 2012

Surgery of the Nose and Paranasal Sinuses: Principles and Concepts
Orrett Ogle, DDS and Harry Dym, DDS,
Guest Editors

RECENT ISSUES

May 2011

Dental Implants
Ole T. Jensen, DDS, MS,
Guest Editor

February 2011

Reoperative Oral and Maxillofacial Surgery
Luis G. Vega, DDS and
Rui Fernandes, DMD, MD,
Guest Editors

November 2010

Psychological Issues for the Oral and Maxillofacial Surgeon
Hillel Ephros, DMD, MD,
Guest Editor

RELATED INTEREST

Atlas of the Oral and Maxillofacial Surgery Clinics of North America,
March 2011 (Vol. 19, No. 1)
Peripheral Trigeminal Nerve Injury, Repair, and Regeneration
Martin B. Steed, DDS, *Guest Editor*

THE CLINICS ARE NOW AVAILABLE ONLINE!
Access your subscription at:
www.theclinics.com

Preface
Complications in Dentoalveolar Surgery

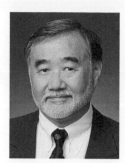
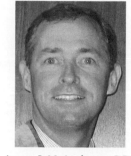

Dennis-Duke R. Yamashita, DDS   James P. McAndrews, DDS
Guest Editors

The responsibility of the oral and maxillofacial surgeon is to provide the best possible result for their patients. In today's society, the barometer of success does not end at a successful surgery, but in the ultimate achievement of the clinician's goals as well as those of the patient. The scope of our specialty is vast, ranging from dentoalveolar procedures and trauma management to cosmetic and reconstructive surgery. Yet, for most of us, the core of our practice remains dentoalveolar surgery. While we have developed the most advanced surgical methods and techniques, it is the management and treatment of complications that will continue to be the most challenging aspects of our practices.

This issue attempts to address some of the medical and surgical complications that may be encountered during the care and treatment of our patients. We asked our contributors to dedicate their efforts to producing a work that would inform and educate the reader about some of the common and less common perils related to dentoalveolar surgery. In our opinion, the authors have excelled in this pursuit. The articles in this issue review various problems and offer practical guidelines for successful management.

The complications related to surgical misadventures, nerve injury, hemostasis, local anesthesia, and grafting are reviewed, as well as the surgical and medical management of dentoalveolar infec-

tions, osteoradionecrosis, and bisphosphonate-related necrosis. The issue concludes with a discussion of the failure to diagnose issues as they relate to pathology and the medico-legal aspects associated with dentoalveolar complications.

We would like to thank our contributors, who have shared with us their vast knowledge and experience in this issue. It is through their collective wisdom that we may enhance our decision-making process and thus ensure the highest quality of care for our patients. The practice of oral and maxillofacial surgery will inevitably result in complications, but we hope this issue will serve as a valuable tool in their prevention or management. We wish to express our special thanks to Ms Julie Yamashita for her review of our manuscripts.

Dennis-Duke R. Yamashita, DDS
James P. McAndrews, DDS

Oral and Maxillofacial Surgery
Department of Dentistry
Los Angeles County/USC Medical Center
1100 North State Street, A3C
Los Angeles, CA 90033, USA

E-mail addresses:
dyamashi@usc.edu (D-D.R. Yamashita)
jmcandre@usc.edu (J.P. McAndrews)

Oral Maxillofacial Surg Clin N Am 23 (2011) ix
doi:10.1016/j.coms.2011.05.002
1042-3699/11/$ – see front matter © 2011 Elsevier Inc. All rights reserved.

Complications of Local Anesthesia Used in Oral and Maxillofacial Surgery

David R. Cummings, DDS[a,b],
Dennis-Duke R. Yamashita, DDS, FACD, FICD[c,*],
James P. McAndrews, DDS, FACD, FICD[c]

KEYWORDS

- Local anesthesia • Complications • Dental • Lidocaine
- Paresthesia • Ocular • Toxicity • Articaine

Local anesthetics are used routinely in oral and maxillofacial surgery. Local anesthetics are safe and effective drugs but do have risks that practitioners need to be aware of. This article reviews the complications of local anesthesia. A brief history is provided and the regional and systemic complications that can arise from using local anesthesia are discussed. These complications include paresthesia, ocular complications, allergies, toxicity, and methemoglobinemia. Understanding the risks involved with local anesthesia decreases the chances of adverse events occurring and ultimately leads to improved patient care.

HISTORY OF LOCAL ANESTHESIA

In the 1860s, the first local anesthetic was isolated from coca leaves by Albert Niemann in Germany. Twenty years later, Sigmund Freud was researching the body's ability to adapt to adverse circumstances. Freud had ordered some coca leaves and chewed them, only to find out that they made his tongue numb. Freud had a young colleague who was an ophthalmology resident, by the name of Karl Koller. Freud suggested that Koller try cocaine as a local anesthetic. In 1884, Koller published the first paper on the use of cocaine as a local anesthetic agent. He placed a 2% cocaine solution onto the corneas of rabbits and dogs, causing insensitivity to painful stimuli.[1] Following Koller's work, Halsted administered cocaine near the mandibular nerve of a medical student, and within a few minutes, the student's tongue, lower lip, and teeth were numb. Halsted went on to become a world-renowned professor of surgery at the Johns Hopkins University and is credited as the discoverer of conduction anesthesia. Soon after, the Harrison Narcotics Tax Act outlawed the sale and distribution of cocaine in the United States. In 1905, another important advance in local anesthesia occurred: the discovery of procaine (Novocain) by Alfred Einhorn.[2]

The authors have nothing to disclose.
a Department of Oral and Maxillofacial Surgery, University of Southern California School of Dentistry, Los Angeles County/University of Southern California Medical Center, 925 West 34th Street, Los Angeles, CA 90089, USA
b Private Practice, 26302 La Paz Suite 102, Mission Viejo, CA 92691, USA
c Oral and Maxillofacial Surgery, Department of Dentistry, Los Angeles County/University of Southern California Medical Center, 1100 North State Street, A3C, Los Angeles, CA 90033
* Corresponding author. Oral and Maxillofacial Surgery, Department of Dentistry, Los Angeles County/University of Southern California Medical Center, 1100 North State Street, A3C, Los Angeles, CA 90033.
E-mail address: dyamashi@usc.edu

Oral Maxillofacial Surg Clin N Am 23 (2011) 369–377
doi:10.1016/j.coms.2011.04.009
1042-3699/11/$ – see front matter © 2011 Elsevier Inc. All rights reserved.

Soon after, adrenaline was added to procaine to increase its efficacy. In 1949, a Swedish company introduced lidocaine, an amino amide–based local anesthetic that had fewer side effects and provided a deeper anesthetic compared with Novocain. In 2000, the US Food and Drug Administration approved articaine 4% with epinephrine 1:100,000, and articaine 4% with epinephrine 1:200,000. Lidocaine is currently the most widely used local dental anesthetic in most countries.[3]

REGIONAL COMPLICATIONS
Paresthesia

The incidence of paresthesia after inferior alveolar nerve block has been reported by Pogrel to be as low at 1:850,000 and as high as 1:20,000.[4] Others have reported the incidence to be in the range of 0.15% to 0.54% for temporary paresthesia and a range of 0.0001% to 0.01% for permanent paresthesia.[5–8] According to Pogrel and Thamby,[9] there is no statistical difference between the right and left sides when administering a mandibular block, and they also reported a higher incidence of occurrences with the lingual nerve (79%) than with the inferior alveolar nerve (21%).[9] The investigators accounted for this because the mouth is open wide and the lingual nerve is more taut, making the nerve more immobile in the tissue and therefore unable to be deflected by the needle.[9] In 2003, Pogrel[10] studied the lingual nerve in 12 cadavers. Histologically, it was noted that there are from 1 to 8 fascicles making up the lingual nerve. Of the 12 nerves, 4 had only 1 fascicle. It is speculated that a unifascicular nerve may be injured more easily than a multifascicular one. This concept of the unifascicular nerve seems to be the most reasonable explanation for predilection of the lingual nerve compared with the inferior alveolar nerve.

According to Hillerup and Jensen,[11] there is a higher female predilection (67% vs 33%). Kraft and Hickel reported a ratio of women to men only slightly higher than 1:1.[8,12] It is thought that this higher incidence is because women tend to seek more medical care than men. Further investigation is needed in this area.

There are many theories as to the cause of paresthesia following inferior alveolar nerve blocks. Needle trauma, the volume of solution injected, repeated injections, the type of local anesthesia administered, and neurotoxicity are the most commonly reported causes in the literature.

Most practitioners have had patients who have experienced the feeling of an electrical shock at the time of injection, and some practitioners have thought that this is related to the injection injury.

Kraft and Hickel[8] reported an incidence of 7% of this electrical shock occurring at the time of a mandibular block with none of the patients experiencing any nerve injury. With lingual paresthesia, Hillerup and Jensen[11] reported an incidence as high as 40% and found no difference in the severity of nerve injury in patients who had reported feeling an electrical shock compared with those who did not feel the shock. This being said, the sensation was not seen as an indicator of nerve injury. The volume of injection and repeated injections have not been associated with the severity of nerve injury.

There have been reports of increased incidence of paresthesias associated with certain types of local anesthetics when performing inferior alveolar nerve blocks. In 1995, Haas and Lennon[6] reported a 21-year retrospective study on paresthesias after administration of local anesthesia. The investigators reported 143 cases of paresthesia following mandibular blocks in which no surgical procedures were performed. In most of these cases, the patients received the standard volume of solution of 1.8 mL. The frequency of paresthesia was found to be 33.6% for articaine, 3.4% for lidocaine, 4% for mepivacaine, 43% for prilocaine, and 47% for unknown causes. These numbers are based on an estimated use of these drugs in Ontario, Canada, at that time.[13] The investigators believed that their studies supported the concept that local anesthetics do have the potential for neurotoxicity and that there was a higher incidence with articaine and prilocaine. These investigators also did a follow-up study between 1994 and 1998, and their conclusions were the same, showing again that prilocaine and articaine were more commonly associated with paresthesias than any other local anesthetic.

In 2001, Malamed and colleagues[14] published 3 identical single-dose, randomized, double-blinded, parallel-group, active-controlled multicenter study. The investigators reported on 882 injections of 4% articaine with epinephrine 1:100,000, and 443 injections of 2% lidocaine with epinephrine 1:100,000. The incidence of paresthesia was 0.9% and hypesthesia was 0.7% with articaine. The incidence for lidocaine was 0.45% paresthesia and 0.2% hypesthesia. Malamed and colleagues[14] concluded that 4% articaine with epinephrine is an effective anesthetic with a low risk of toxicity that seems comparable with that of other local anesthetics.

Hillerup and Jensen[11] reported on 54 patients with 52 injuries from inferior alveolar nerve blocks. The distribution of paresthesia with specific local anesthesia was as follows: articaine, 54%; prilocaine, 19%; lidocaine, 19%; mepivacaine, 7%, and mepivacaine plus articaine, 1%. The concentrations of these local anesthetics were as follows: articaine, 4%; prilocaine, 3%; lidocaine, 2%; and mepivacaine, 3%. The investigators found an increase in the number of patients with injection injuries after the introduction of articaine 4% into the Danish market. The investigators suggested that since the introduction of articaine in 2000, there was no increase in the use of inferior alveolar nerve blocks but they did state that they did not have precise data to support this assumption. Until more information becomes available, another agent should be considered when clinicians are administering inferior alveolar nerve blocks.

In 2007, Pogrel[4] published his report on 57 patients who were referred to him for evaluation of paresthesia that could have only resulted from an inferior alveolar nerve block. None of these patients underwent any surgical procedures. The numbers of cases reported were as follows: 20 cases of lidocaine, 17 cases of prilocaine, 17 cases of articaine, 1 case of lidocaine and prilocaine, 1 case of prilocaine and lidocaine, and 1 case of bupivacaine. The percentage of sales per year reported by Pogrel at that time was 54% lidocaine, 6% prilocaine, 25% articaine, and 15% mepivacaine. The relative sales of cartridges per year in the United States at that time was the predominant reason for Pogrel submitting his paper because he did not want to find that, although sales figures remained high for articaine, it was not being used for inferior alveolar nerve blocks. Pogrel was confident that this was not taking place in his area. Based on this assumption, he did not see any disproportionate nerve involvement from the use of articaine.

Garisto and colleagues[15] recently published a review of all cases of paresthesia reported to the US Food and Drug Administration Adverse Event Reporting System between 1997 and 2008. The investigators found 226 cases in which only 1 local anesthetic agent was used and nonsurgical dentistry was performed. Of these, 4% articaine was found to be involved in 116 cases (51.3%), 4% prilocaine in 97 cases (42.9%), 2% lidocaine in 11 cases (4.9%), 0.5% bupivacaine in 1 case (0.4%), and 3% mepivacaine in 1 case (0.4%).[15] These results were consistent with the reports from Canada and Denmark.[6,11,16] The investigators corroborated the earlier findings that suggested that the use of prilocaine and articaine, either alone or in combination, may be associated with an increased risk of developing paresthesia.[6,9,11,16–18] The investigators noted that articaine and prilocaine are the only dental local anesthetics formulated as 4% solutions in the United States; all others are at lower concentrations.

In 2009, Gaffen and Haas[17] reviewed all nonsurgical paresthesias reported to the Ontario Professional Liability Program from 1999 to 2008 inclusively. They found the mean age to be 43.8 years with a higher proportion of women (51.1%) than for men (48.9%) were affected. They found that the tongue was affected more often than the lip and chin (79.1% and 28%, respectively). During this period, there were 147 cases reported. Articaine alone was associated with 109 cases (59.9%) of paresthesia, prilocaine with 29 cases (15.9%), lidocaine with 23 cases (12.6%), and mepivacaine with 6 cases (3.3%), and no cases of bupivacaine alone were reported. The investigators state that their data are not perfect. They noted that it is difficult to get approval for prospective experimental designs from institutional review boards and that the incidence of paresthesia is based on assumptions of the frequency of mandibular blocks used. Thus, the reported incidence should be viewed cautiously. Their results indicate that articaine and prilocaine are associated with reporting rates of nonsurgical paresthesia that are significantly higher than expected based on the rate of use of these drugs. Notably, these local anesthetics are available in dental cartridges in Canada solely as 4% solutions. Gaffen and Haas[17] suggested that it is not the drug per se but the higher dose of the drug combined with the mechanical insult that predisposes the nerve to permanent damage.

What causes paresthesia after the administration of local anesthesia remains unclear. The most common theories are direct trauma to the nerve, intraneural hematoma, or potential neurotoxicity from the local anesthetic itself.[11,15,17] Needle breakage has been covered in another article in this issue (see the article by Alexander and Attia elsewhere in this issue for further exploration of this topic). High concentrations of local anesthetics have been shown to result in an irreversible conduction block of 5% lidocaine versus 1.5% lidocaine in a study by Lambert and colleagues.[19] Histologically, studies have primarily supported this theory; one study using microinjections in rat sciatic and cat lingual nerves showed no significant effect.[20–22] Proposed mechanisms for this irreversible nerve injury are membrane disruption, characteristic of a detergent effect, and that local anesthetic neurotoxicity relates to their octanol/buffer coefficients. An assessment of apoptosis (programmed cell death) induced by different local anesthetics on neuroblastoma cell lines also demonstrates this dose-response relationship of local anesthetics. The in vitro findings indicated that all local anesthetics induced dose-dependent apoptosis. This study also determined that, at the anesthetic concentrations used in dentistry, only prilocaine, but not articaine, was more neurotoxic than lidocaine.[23] More studies are needed to further understand the cause of this rare adverse complication.

Ocular Complications

There have been many different reports of ocular complications following the administration of local anesthesia for dentistry. Signs and symptoms including tissue blanching, hematoma formation, facial paralysis, diplopia, amaurosis, ptosis, mydriasis, miosis, enophthalmos, and even permanent blindness have been reported.

Blanching of the tissue over the skin of the injection site can occur but this disappears as the drug is absorbed into the systemic circulation. Blanching can occur as a result of the contraction of the blood vessel in reaction to the impact or by mechanical stimulation of sympathetic vasoconstrictor fibers supplying the area. The management of this is supportive, and symptoms resolve quickly.[24] Facial nerve paralysis is most commonly caused by the introduction of local anesthetics into the capsule of the parotid gland. The nerve trunk of the facial nerve is located at the posterior border of the ramus of the mandible, and directing the needle posteriorly or overinsertion can place the needle into this area when performing an inferior alveolar nerve block. This complication leads to the inability to close the ipsilateral eye, but the corneal reflex is still intact. The duration of the paralysis depends on the duration of action of that specific local anesthetic, which is generally only a few hours, and supportive management is usually all that is needed.[25]

Diplopia following administration of local anesthesia for dental procedures is an uncommon complication, but does occur.[26–31] The cause is not clear, but the most common theory is back pressure from an inferior alveolar nerve block traveling back into the maxillary artery via retrograde flow and gaining access into the middle meningeal artery to the ophthalmic artery, which causes the symptoms, such as diplopia, to appear.[32] Furthermore, in 4% of patients, the ophthalmic artery is established not from the internal carotid artery but from the middle meningeal artery, which follows uninterrupted flow from the external carotid artery.[33] These symptoms usually resolve with time, lasting from a few minutes to a few hours.[34]

Horner-like syndrome has also been reported following the administration of local anesthesia for dentistry.[34,35] This syndrome involves mydriasis, ptosis, and diplopia. According to Ngeow and colleagues,[35] this condition is caused by a sympathetic block at the ciliary ganglion once the anesthetic solution reaches the ganglion. Campbell and colleagues[36] believed that this theory was illogical because of the considerable anatomic distance involved and that a sympathetic block would induce much broader symptoms not seen in these cases. In 1972, Rood[37] had described the arterial route discussed earlier in this article. According to his theory, the vasoconstrictive agent traveled via the inferior alveolar artery back to the maxillary artery to the middle meningeal artery. From the middle meningeal artery, the agent traveled to the lacrimal artery and then via anastomotic connections to the ophthalmic artery. The arteries nurturing the extrinsic and intrinsic muscles of the eye developed vasoconstriction.

Kronman and Kabani[26] proposed that in perivascular trauma, the intra-arterial injection stimulates the sympathetic fibers running alongside the internal maxillary artery until it reaches the orbit, which would account for the vasoconstriction and mydriasis. There is also a local diffusion phenomenon communicating with the pterygoid venous plexus and the ophthalmic vein through the orbital fissure.[30,31] Goldenberg[28] also described that local anesthetic could pass through the cavernous sinus toward the ophthalmic vein, ultimately reaching the ophthalmic artery by way of a series of anastomoses.

Amaurosis is vision loss or weakness that occurs without an apparent lesion affecting the eye. This condition has been reported often in the literature following the administration of local anesthesia for dental procedures. Boynes[38] reviewed the literature from 1957 to 2010 and found 48 cases of ocular complications, and of those, 9 cases of amaurosis were reported. Rishiraj and colleagues reported a patient with permanent vision loss in one eye following the administration of local anesthesia for a dental extraction.[39,40] Wilke[41] claimed that instantaneous blindness results from the anesthetic agent being carried into the central artery of the retina through the anastomosis of the ophthalmic and middle meningeal arteries via the recurrent meningeal branch of the lacrimal artery. Also included in the differential diagnosis are emboli of the ophthalmic artery, reflex vascular spasm, oil emboli, toxic action on retinal cells, chronic inflammation, and generation of a thrombus from vascular trauma.[24,39] The mechanism of action is not fully understood at this time; so until this is discovered, it is important that when this condition occurs, the patient is reassured that symptoms are typically transient. When ocular complications persist, an ophthalmology consultation is prudent. Aspiration at the time of administration of local anesthesia is very important and minimizes the risk of ocular complications.

Trismus, Pain, and Infection

Trismus is a term used to describe limited movement of the mandible. Postinjection trismus can and does occur after the administration of local anesthesia for inferior alveolar blocks. This condition can be caused by hematoma, infection, multiple injections, excessive volume of local anesthetics, and sterilizing solutions that can potentially cause trismus. Management usually consists of moist heat, antiinflammatory agents, and range of motion excercises.[25] Most cases resolve within 6 weeks, with a range of 4 to 20 weeks.[3]

Pain from the delivery of local anesthesia can be caused by rapid delivery of the solution into the tissue by a dull needle from multiple injections and barbed needles at the time the needle is withdrawn.

Contamination of a needle is the major cause of infection after the administration of local anesthesia. This situation rarely occurs with the use of sterile disposable needles and aseptically stored glass cartridges.[25] Odontogenic infections are covered in another article in this issue (see the article by Lypka and Hammoudeh elsewhere in this issue for further exploration of this topic).

Malamed[25] suggests the following to help prevent infection from occurring: use proper techniques, use a sharp needle, use proper topical anesthesia, use sterile local anesthetics, inject slowly, and use a solution that is at room temperature.

SYSTEMIC COMPLICATIONS
Allergic Reactions

Allergic reactions due to the administration of local anesthesia are uncommon but can occur. The incidence of true allergies to amide local anesthetics is widely accepted to be less than 1%.[42] In the 1980s, methylparaben was removed from the market. Methylparaben was a preservative used to increase the shelf life of local anesthetics. Before this, most allergic reactions were associated with procaine. The antigenicity of procaine and other ester agents is most often related to the para-aminobenzoic acid component of ester anesthetics, a decidedly antigenic compound.[43] Adverse reactions caused by fear and anxiety, inadvertent intravascular administration of local anesthetic, toxic overdose, intolerance, and idiosyncrasy can be mistaken for a true allergic response.[44] There are a few different tests that can be used by the allergist to document an allergy to local anesthesia, such as the skin prick test, the interdermal or subcutaneous placements test, and/or the drug provocative challenge test. Most allergists consider the drug provocative test to be the gold standard in the diagnosis of drug allergy.[45] Allergies to local anesthetic may be type I or type IV hypersensitivity reactions, with the type I response more commonly reported.[46–48]

Sulfites are commonly used to extend the shelf life of local anesthetics. Sulfites are antioxidants that help stabilize the epinephrine in the local anesthetic solution.[9] The most common sulfites used currently are metabisulfite, sodium bisulfate, and potassium bisulfite. Local anesthetics containing vasoconstrictors should be used cautiously or withheld in patients reporting food allergies associated with sulfites.[49] In these situations, formulations of local anesthesia that do not contain vasoconstrictors are recommended, such as 3% mepivacaine or 4% prilocaine.

Most types of allergic reactions that concern practitioners are type I (anaphylactoid). Signs and symptoms include skin manifestations (erythema, pruritus, urticaria), gastrointestinal manifestations (muscle cramping, nausea and vomiting, incontinence), respiratory manifestations (coughing, wheezing, dyspnea, laryngeal edema), and cardiovascular manifestations (palpitations, tachycardia, hypotension, unconsciousness, cardiac arrest).[50] Treatment of allergic reactions depends on the severity of the reaction. Mild forms are usually managed by oral or intramuscular antihistamines, such as diphenhydramine, 25 to 50 mg. If serious signs or symptoms develop, immediate treatment becomes necessary, and this includes basic life support, intramuscular or subcutaneous epinephrine 0.3 to 0.5 mg, and activating the emergency response system for transportation to the local hospital for acute therapy.[51]

Toxicity

Reactions from local anesthesia are infrequent, and when properly treated, they are unlikely to result in significant morbidity or mortality. Toxicity can be caused by excessive dosing of either the local anesthetic or the vasoconstrictor. When local anesthesia is given, some of it diffuses away from the injection site into the systemic circulation where it is metabolized and eliminated. Blood levels of either the vasoconstrictor or the local anesthetic increase if there is an inadvertent intravascular injection, if there are repeated injections of the local anesthetic, or if excessive volumes are used in pediatric dentistry. The addition of the vasoconstrictor is used to reduce the absorption systemically.[52]

Adhering to local anesthetic dosing guidelines is one of the most important factors in the prevention of toxicity. Local anesthetic dosing guidelines are based on the type of local anesthetic agent used

Table 1
The maximum recommended doses of injectable local anesthetics

Agents (Brand Name)	Concentration of Local Anesthetic		Concentration of Epi/Levo	Maximum Dosing		Maximum Number of Cartridges		
	mg/mL[a]	mg/Cartridge[b]	mg/Cartridge[c]	Adult MRD (mg)	MRD/lb[d] (mg/lb)	Adults[e]	50-lb Child	25-lb Child
2% lidocaine, 1:100,000 epi	20	36	0.018	500	3.3	13.8	4.6	2.3
2% lidocaine, 1:50,000 epi	20	36	0.036	500	3.3	13.8	4.6	2.3
2% lidocaine, plain	20	36	—	300	2.0	8.3	2.8	1.4
4% articaine, 1:100,000 epi	40	72	0.018[e]	500	3.3	6.9	2.3	1.1
4% articaine, 1:200,000 epi	40	72	0.009[e]	500	3.3	6.9	2.3	1.1
3% mepivacaine	30	54	—	400	2.6	7.4	2.5	1.2
2% mepivacaine, 1:20,000 levo	20	36	0.09	400	2.6	11.1	3.7	1.8
4% prilocaine	40	72	—	600	4.0	8.3	2.8	1.4
4% prilocaine, 1:200,000 epi	40	72	0.009	600	4.0	8.3	2.8	1.4
0.5% bupivacaine, 1:200,000 epi	5	9	0.009	90	0.6	10	NR	NR

All cartridges are assumed to contain approximately 1.8 mL.

Abbreviations: epi, epinephrine; levo, levonordefrin; MRD, maximum recommended dose; NR, not recommended.

[a] Calculation for drug concentration: for example, 2% lidocaine solution = 2 g/100 mL = 2000 mg/100 mL = 20 mg/mL.

[b] Calculation of mg/cartridge: for example, 2% lidocaine: 20 mg/mL × 1.8 mL/cartridge = 36 mg/cartridge.

[c] Calculation of mg/cartridge of epinephrine: for example, 1:100,000 mL = 0.01 mg/mL = 100,000 mL = 1 g; 100,000 mL = 1000 mg; 100,000 mL = 0.018 mg of epi. A 1.8-mL cartridge contains 0.018 mg of epi.

[d] Calculation of weight-based MRD: for example, 500 mg for a 150-lb adult = 500 mg/150 lb = 3.3 mg/lb.

[e] Calculation of maximum number of cartridges: for example, for lidocaine/epinephrine, the adult MRD for lidocaine/epi is 500 mg; 500 mg/36 mg per cartridge = 13.8 cartridges.

From Moore PA, Hersh EV. Local anesthetics: pharmacology and toxicity. Dent Clin North Am 2010;54(4):593; with permission.

and the weight of the patient. Dosing is most critical in the pediatric population because the pediatric patient weighs less, and the dose must be lowered. Clark's rule is used when treating pediatric patients. The formula is child's dose = (child's weight/adult weight) × (adult dose).[52] Another simple way to calculate maximum safe dosages for all anesthetic formulations used in dentistry is called the rule of 25, which states that a dentist may safely use 1 cartridge of any local anesthetic for every 11.4 kg (25 lbs) of patient weight.[51] **Table 1** shows the maximum recommended dosages published by Moore and Hersh.[52]

The local anesthetic mepivacaine plain has been associated with numerous reports of toxicity.[53,54] This local anesthetic has no vasoconstrictor and comes in a 3% solution. The lack of vasoconstrictor leads to increased systemic absorption, and with a higher concentration of solution, it shows a higher probability of the local anesthetic being absorbed into circulation. Toxicity from local anesthesia usually starts with an excitatory phase, which maybe be brief or may not occur at all.[25] The excitatory phase, when it does occur, can manifest as tremors, muscle twitching, shivering, and clonic tonic convulsions. This phase is followed by generalized central nervous system depression and possible life-threatening respiratory depression. With extremely high doses, cardiac excitability and cardiac conduction decrease. The cardiac manifestations include ectopic rhythms, bradycardia and ensuing peripheral vasodilation, and significant hypotension. Treatment should address respiratory depression and convulsions. Vital signs should be monitored, the airway maintained, basic life support administered, and the emergency medical support services should be called. Intravenous diazepam or midazolam may be administered for a seizure that does not seem to be stopping.[25]

Methemoglobinemia

Methemoglobinemia is a reaction that can occur after administration of amide local anesthetics, nitrates, and aniline dyes. Prilocaine and benzocaine are used in dentistry and may induce methemoglobinemia. Methemoglobinemia occurs when the iron atom within the hemoglobin molecule is oxidized. The iron atom goes from a ferrous state to a ferric state. Once the hemoglobin molecule is in the ferric state, it is referred to as methemoglobin. Physiologically, the hemoglobin molecule cannot deliver as much oxygen to the tissue because of its increased affinity for its bound oxygen and its decreased affinity for unbound oxygen.[55] Drugs used in dentistry and oral and maxillofacial surgery that have been implicated include prilocaine, benzocaine, EMLA (eutectic mixture local anesthetic) cream, and nitrous oxide. There are 2 metabolites of prilocaine that are responsible for the oxidation of hemoglobin.[56]

Benzocaine is a topical anesthetic that can be used before local anesthetic injections, before taking radiographs as a topical gel, and as a spray before direct laryngoscopy. Benzocaine is a well-documented but poorly understood cause of methemoglobinemia. EMLA cream is a product containing prilocaine and lidocaine. The final product contains 2.5% prilocaine in the cream. The product is designed to be applied to the skin but it has also been used to anesthetize the gingiva for deep cleaning. The maximum amount to be applied is 5 applicators (212 mg) of prilocaine.

There have been a few articles published linking nitrous oxide to metahemoglobinemia.[51,57] After a critical review of these articles, Trapp and Will[55] concluded from these 2 articles that there is no compelling evidence for the role of nitrous oxide as an oxidant of hemoglobin.

Signs and symptoms usually do not appear for 3 to 4 hours after the administration of large doses of local anesthesia.[25] Clinical signs of cyanosis are observed when blood levels of methemoglobin reach 10% to 20%, and dyspnea and tachycardia are observed when methemoglobin levels reach 35% to 40%.[57] The diagnosis is made by a blood sample and a co-oximetry test. In 2005, the Rainbow Rad57 was introduced as a noninvasive method to measure methemoglobin levels.[55] Co-oximetry is a conventional pulse oximetry that also measures the methemoglobin and carboxyhemoglobin levels. Methylene blue 1 to 2 mg/kg intravenously is used for the treatment of methemoglobinemia.

SUMMARY

Local anesthetics are a routine part in all oral and maxillofacial practices. These drugs are safe and effective but do have inherent risks. Most of the complications discussed are rare but can and do occur. Minimizing adverse outcomes is the goal of all practitioners. This goal can be accomplished by using the appropriate local anesthetics in certain situations (patient allergies), calculating dosages to help prevent toxicity, and aspirating while giving local anesthesia to help prevent local and/or systemic complications. These techniques are important for any dentist to minimize adverse outcomes when administering local anesthesia.

REFERENCES

1. Ring ME. The history of local anesthesia. J Calif Dent Assoc 2007;35(4):275–82.
2. Wawersik J. History of anesthesia in Germany. J Clin Anesth 1991;3(3).235–44.
3. Center for Drug Evaluation and Research. Approved drug products with therapeutic equivalence evaluations. 27th edition. Washington, DC: US Food and Drug Administration; 2007.
4. Pogrel MA. Permanent nerve damage from inferior alveolar nerve blocks—an update to include articaine. J Calif Dent Assoc 2007;35(4):271–3.
5. Paxton K, Thome DE. Efficacy of articaine formulations: quantitative reviews. Dent Clin North Am 2010;54(4):643–53.
6. Haas DA, Lennon D. A 21 year retrospective study of reports of paresthesia following local anesthetic administration. J Can Dent Assoc 1995; 61:319–30.
7. Harn SD, Durham TM. Incidence of lingual nerve trauma and post injection complications in conventional mandibular block anesthesia. J Am Dent Assoc 1990;121:519–23.
8. Kraft TC, Hickel R. Clinical investigation into the incidence of direct damage to the lingual nerve caused by local anesthesia. J Craniomaxillofac Surg 1994; 22:294–6.
9. Pogrel MA, Thamby S. Permanent nerve involvement resulting from inferior alveolar nerve blocks. J Am Dent Assoc 2004;131:901–7.
10. Pogrel MA, Schmidt BL, Sambajon V, et al. Lingual nerve damage due to inferior alveolar nerve blocks: a possible explanation. J Am Dent Assoc 2003; 134(2):195–9.
11. Hillerup S, Jensen R. Nerve injury caused by mandibular block analgesia. Int J Oral Maxillofac Surg 2006;35:437–43.
12. Cornelius CP, Roser M, Wietholter H, et al. Nerve injection injuries due to local anesthetics. Experimental work. J Craniomaxillofac Surg 2000; 28(Suppl 3):134–5.
13. Haas DA, Lennon D. Local anesthetic use by dentists in Ontario. J Can Dent Assoc 1995;61:297–304.
14. Malamed SF, Gagnon S, Lebalanc D. Articaine hydrochloride: a study of the safety of a new amide local anesthetic. J Am Dent Assoc 2001;132:177–85.
15. Garisto GA, Gaffen AS, Lawrence HP, et al. Occurrence of paresthesia after dental local anesthetic administration in the United States. J Am Dent Assoc 2010;141(7):836–44.
16. Miller PA, Haas DA. Incidence of local anesthetic-induced neuropathies in Ontario form 1994–1998. [abstract]. J Dent Res 2000;79:62.
17. Gaffen AS, Haas DA. Retrospective review of voluntary reports of nonsurgical paresthesia in dentistry. J Can Dent Assoc 2009;75(8).579.

18. Legarth J. Skader pa nervus lingualis opstaet i forbindelse med mandibularanalgesi: anmeldt til Dansk Tandlaegeforenings Patientskadeforsikring 2002–2004. Tandlaegebladet 2005;109(10):786–8 [in Danish].
19. Lambert LA, Lambert DH, Strichartz GR. Irreversible conduction block in isolated nerve by high concentrations of local anesthetics. Anesthesiology 1994; 80:1082–93.
20. Kalichman MW, Powell HC, Myers RR. Quantitative histologic analysis of local anesthetic-induced injury to rat sciatic nerve. J Pharmacol Exp Ther 1989;250: 406–13.
21. Kalichman MW. Physiologic mechanisms by which local anesthetics may cause injury to nerve and spinal cord. Reg Anesth 1993;18:448–52.
22. Hoffmeister B. Morphologic veranderungen peripherer nerven nach intraneuraler lokal anasthesie injektion. Dtsch Zahnarztl Z 1991;46:828 [in German].
23. Moore PA, Haas DA. Paresthesias in dentistry. Dent Clin North Am 2010;54(4):715–30.
24. Uckan S, Cilasun U, Erkman O. Rare ocular and cutaneous complication of inferior alveolar nerve block. J Oral Maxillofac Surg 2006;64:719–21.
25. Malamed SF. Handbook of local anesthesia. 5th edition. Philadelphia: Elsevier Mosby; 2004.
26. Kronman JH, Kabani S. The neuronal basis for diplopia following local anesthetic injections. Oral Surg Oral Med Oral Pathol 1984;58:533–4.
27. Goldenberg AS. Transient diplopia from a posterior alveolar injection. J Endod 1990;16:550–1.
28. Goldenberg AS. Diplopia resulting from a mandibular injection. J Endod 1983;9:261–2.
29. Petrelli A, Steller RE. Medial rectus muscle palsy after dental anesthesia. Am J Ophthalmol 1980;90:422–4.
30. Marinho RM. Abducent nerve palsy following dental local analgesia. Br Dent J 1995;179:69–70.
31. Hyams SW. Oculomotor palsy following dental anesthesia. Arch Ophthalmol 1976;94:1281.
32. Choi EH, Seo JY, Jung BY, et al. Diplopia after inferior alveolar nerve block anesthesia: report of 2 cases and literature review. Oral Surg Oral Med Oral Pathol 2009;107:e21–4.
33. Singh S, Dass R. The central artery of the retina. I. Origin and course. Br J Ophthalmol 1960;44:193–212.
34. Diago PM, Bielsa JM. Ophthalmologic complications after intraoral local anesthesia with articaine. Oral Surg Oral Med Oral Pathol 2000;90:21–4.
35. Ngeow WC, Shim CK, Chai WL. Transient loss of power of accommodation in one eye following inferior alveolar nerve block: report of two cases. J Can Dent Assoc 2006;72:927–31.
36. Campbell RL, Mercuri LG, van Sickels J. Cervical sympathetic block following intraoral local anesthesia. Oral Surg Oral Med Oral Pathol 1979;47: 223–6.

37. Rood JP. Ocular complication of inferior dental nerve block. A case report. Br Dent J 1972;132:23–4.

38. Boynes S, Echeverria Z, Abdulwahab M. Ocular complications associated with local anesthesia administered in dentistry. Dent Clin N Am 2010;54:677–86.

39. Rishiraj B, Epstein JB, Fine D, et al. Permanent vision loss in one eye following administration of local anesthesia for a dental extraction. Int J Oral Maxillofac Surg 2005;34(2):220–3.

40. Hinton RJ, Dechow C, Carlson DS. Recovery of jaw muscle function following injection of a myotoxic agent (lidocaine-epinephrine). Oral Surg Oral Med Oral Pathol 1985;59(3):247–51.

41. Wilke GJ. Temporary uniocular blindness and ophthalmoplegia associated with a mandibular block injection. A case report. Aust Dent J 2000;45:131.

42. Giovannitti JA, Bennett CR. Assessment of allergy to local anesthetics. J Am Dent Assoc 1979;98:701–9.

43. Miller RD, Stoelting RK. Basics of anesthesia. 5th edition. Philadelphia: Churchill Livingstone; 2007. p. 124–6.

44. Ball IA. Allergic reactions to lignocaine. Braz Dent J 2003;186:224–6.

45. Schorr WP, Mohajerin AH. Paraben sensitivity. Arch Dermatol 1966;93:721–3.

46. Noormalin A, Shahnaz M, Rosmilah M, et al. IgE-mediated hypersensitivity reaction to lidocaine—case report. Trop Biomed 2005;22:179–83.

47. Fuzier R, Lapeyre-Mstre M, Mertes PM, et al. Immediate- and delayed-type allergic reactions to amide local anesthetics: clinical features and skin testing. Pharmacoepidemiol Drug Saf 2009;18:595–601.

48. The Associated Press. FDA plans warning on drugs with sulfites. New York: The New York Times; 1986.

49. Campbell JC, Maestrello CI, Campbell RI. Allergic response to metabisulfite in lidocaine anesthetic solution. Anesth Prog 2001;48:21–6.

50. Speca S, Boynes S, Cuddy M. Allergic reactions to local anesthetic formulations. Dent Clin North Am 2010;54(4):655–64.

51. Finder RL, Moore PA. Adverse drug reactions to local anesthesia. Dent Clin North Am 2002;46:747–57.

52. Moore PA, Hersh EV. Local anesthetics: pharmacology and toxicity. Dent Clin North Am 2010;54(4):587–99.

53. Goodson JM, Moore PA. Life-threatening reactions after pedodontic sedation: an assessment of narcotic, local anesthetic and antiemetic drug interaction. J Am Dent Assoc 1983;107:239–45.

54. Moore PA, Goodson JM. Risk appraisal of narcotic sedation for children. Anesth Prog 1985;32:129–39.

55. Trapp L, Will J. Acquired methemoglobinemia revisited. Dent Clin North Am 2010;54(4):665–75.

56. Vasters FG, Eberhart LH, Koch T, et al. Risk factors for prilocaine-induced methaemoglobinaemia following peripheral regional anesthesia. Eur J Anaesthesiol 2006;23:760–5.

57. Ash-Bernal R, Wise R, Wright SM. Acquired methemoglobinemia: a retrospective series of 138 cases at 2 teaching hospitals. Medicine 2004;83(5):265–73.

Oral Maxillofacial Surgery Displacement Complications

Gerald Alexander, DDS[a,b,c,*], Hany Attia, DDS[b]

KEYWORDS

- Dentoalveolar complications • Maxillofacial complications
- Displaced surgical instrumentation

An iatrogenically displaced object, although seldom anticipated and almost always inadvert, can present a challenge to the primary practitioner or the secondary subsequent surgeon.[1] Though seldom life-threatening, the failure to resolve the problem in a timely fashion can have serious psychological, physiologic, and medical legal consequences. This discussion will emphasize the former and present cases of complications and the resolving treatment. No one sets out to displace an object, whether a tooth, instrument, or ancillary equipment. Of course the paramount issues are anticipation and prevention. When the event occurs, retrieval and repair, whether immediate or delayed, is the task at hand.

Modern imaging techniques can be both helpful and incriminating. Imaging can be as simple as a dental periapical or a panoramic radiograph and be as advanced as a 3-dimensional computed tomography (CT) reconstruction. In-office cone beam 3-dimensional imaging can be beneficial in locating misplaced teeth or foreign objects. Their availability is invaluable and may be, if not already, the standard of care. A chest radiograph or plain abdominal radiograph (KUB) film is often helpful in locating and or documenting negative findings of objects lost beyond the oral cavity. An intraoperative CT in a hospital operating room can be very helpful in an anesthetized patient.

DISPLACED TEETH

Arguably, the most commonly misplaced object in oral maxillofacial surgeries are teeth, both of traumatic or iatrogenic causes. In traumatic losses, unaccounted teeth must be located or, at a minimum, documented of their negative locale. It is not uncommon that trauma patients have loose or unaccounted for traumatically misplaced teeth. It is the duty of the oral maxillofacial surgeon practitioner who evaluates these patients to account for possibly ingested or aspirated teeth via imaging. Imaging previously discussed can help either positively or negatively confirm the location of these lost teeth. If a tooth or object is thought to be lost beyond the oral cavity during an in-office procedure it is prudent to determine whether the object was swallowed or aspirated. If it is obviously aspirated and the patient is in airway distress, a simple finger sweep should first be attempted, followed by a Heimlich procedure. Upper airway aspirations may be retrievable with Magill forceps and the aid of a laryngoscope. If this is not successful, and the patient begins to desaturate, a positive pressure bag connected to an oxygen source can aid in ventilation. If all else fails, intubation or a cricothyroidotomy may be indicated. Transfer of the patient to the emergency room via ambulance should be initiated simultaneously.

The iatrogenic displacement of teeth occurs most frequently in the attempted removal of impacted third molars. It is wise to present this possibility to the patient in the preoperative informed consent discussion. Again anticipation and prevention are key in management of this complication. Common places associated with displaced third molars are the maxillary sinus, temporal space, infratemporal space, lateral

a Private Practice, Fresno, CA, USA
b Department of Oral Maxillofacial Surgery, University of California, San Francisco Fresno, Fresno, CA, USA
c Veterans Affairs Medical Center Fresno, Fresno, CA, USA
* Corresponding author. 7025 North Maple, Suite 108 Fresno, CA 93720.
E-mail address: garunsii@yahoo.com

Oral Maxillofacial Surg Clin N Am 23 (2011) 379–386
doi:10.1016/j.coms.2011.04.001

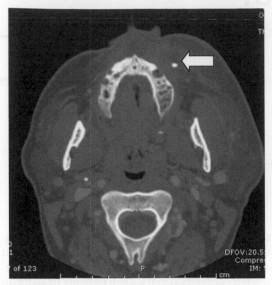

Fig. 1. Root tip lost in the buccal space.

pharyngeal space, submandibular space, and buccal space (**Fig. 1**).

In regards to maxillary third molar complications, if the surgeon is uncomfortable removing an unusually superiorly placed maxillary third molar, then it should be left in place for further eruption. The exception to this would be the presence of any associated or obvious impending pathology.

The most important preventative maneuver is to provide proper access. A high impaction is usually apical and somewhat buccal to the second molar. A preoperative cone beam CT is invaluable in determining the medio–lateral location. If the tooth is apical and reachable from a lateral approach, then enough subperiosteal dissection should be achieved to visualize either a portion of the tooth or its overlying bone. This may require a buccal sulcular incision extending 2 to 3 teeth anteriorly from the maxillary tuberosity or a vertical anterior buccal releasing incision may provide excellent access. Overlying bone is then removed with a mono-beveled osteotome until enough of the impacted tooth is visualized to permit placement of a preferably curved elevator (eg, 190/191 or a pots elevator). The elevator should be placed mesial to the impaction and distal or superiorly to the disto–buccal root of the second molar. The force of the elevation should have a distal and buccal vector. This may require the elevator to engage more than half of the equator of the impacted tooth. This will direct the tooth away from the sinus cavity and the infratemporal space. It may be helpful to place an instrument such as the rounded end of the #9 periosteal elevator distal to the impaction as it is elevated. Controlled force is applied when delivering the impaction. It goes

without saying that a gauze throat pack be appropriately placed to prevent losing the tooth in the posterior pharynx. If the impaction is medial to the second molar and cannot be surgically visualized, it is better left alone than blindly reaching for it.

SINUS DISPLACEMENT

The most commonly associated space with a displaced impacted maxillary third molar is the maxillary sinus. If the impacted tooth or root tip is lost in the maxillary sinus, it is worth trying to visualize the tooth through the site from which it came. Small suction tips may be able to bring the object back into view so that an instrument such as a small hooked scaler or root tip pick can be used to retrieve it. The hole into the sinus may need to be enlarged to suction out the tooth or root tip. If all else fails, a Caldwell luc procedure can be used to access the displaced tooth or root tip (**Fig. 2**A, B). This can be done in the traditional canine fossa approach or through an osteotomy above the second molar. The anterior Caldwell luc approach makes for easier visualization through the osteotomy, as well as easier closure following retrieval of the displaced object. Displaced root tips from other posterior maxillary teeth can also be retrieved in a similar fashion. The patient should be informed of what has occurred and be placed on sinus precautions and appropriate prophylactic antibiotics. In addition to teeth, a poorly planned implant can be lost in the sinus either from iatrogenic forces or physiologic complications (see **Fig. 2**C). In the case of lost implants or other instrumentation for that matter, retrieval can be accomplished with a similar Caldwell luc technique.

Infratemporal Space Displacement

The infratemporal space is also a possible pathway for a displaced maxillary third molar. Its retrieval does not usually present any technical problems once its location is established radiographically. Further displacement of teeth into the temporal fossa may be more technically difficult to access. It is sometimes helpful to place a finger over the temporal area (extraorally) to palpate or stabilize the ectopic tooth while the retrieval is attempted through the extraction site intraorally (Martin Bellenger, DMD, personal communication, 2009). It has also been suggested that by waiting 10 to 14 days, enough fibrous growth will have developed around the tooth to help stabilize the tooth and facilitate its removal.[2]

Another technique that has been described in the literature is to introduce a Kirshner wire lateral to the orbital rim. With bimanual manipulation,

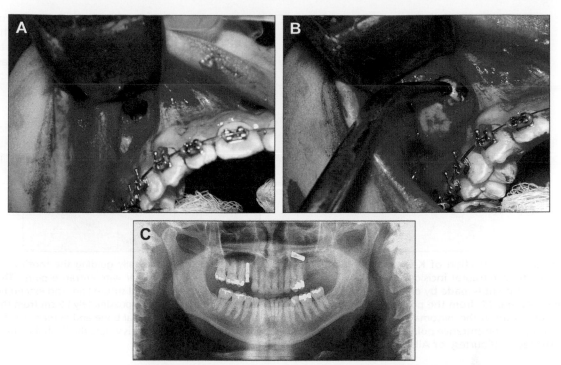

Fig. 2. (*A, B*) Impacted #1 displaced into the maxillary sinus during extraction. View of the tooth through a Caldwell luc approach and removal. (*C*) Panorex showing displaced dental implant in the maxillary sinus.

the Kirshner wire can be guided to the ectopic tooth and pushed back through the extraction site (Allan Malkasian, DDS, personal communication, 2010) (**Fig. 3**).[3] The Kirshner wire should be of a width that can be flexed and, if necessary, a gentle curve be placed at its tip. It is possible that the Kirshner wire may require a blunt end so that it will not slip off the tooth when it is engaged in the temporal fossa. The index finger is placed at the incision site of the third molar socket. The tooth may or may not be palpable at this site. The Kirshner wire is then introduced into the stab incision in the temporal region and passed in a direction that angles toward the third molar socket. For orientation purposes, the Kirshner wire can be extended and used to palpate the maxillary tuberosity, then retracted. At this point the goal is to palpate the tooth with 1 index finger while using the tip (or curved tip) of the Kirshner wire to locate the tooth. When the tooth can be found and palpated with the fingertip, the Kirshner wire is pressed against the tooth, and the index finger is then used as counter pressure against the tooth. While pushing downward with the Kirshner wire and applying counter pressure on the tooth, the tooth is moved downward and out of the temporal fossa. If all else fails, a case report in the literature of a failed removal of a displaced tooth in this area noted that there were no consequences.[4] In addition to

the infratemporal space, a maxillary third molar can uncommonly find its way superiorly along side the condylar head (**Fig. 4**).

Mandibular third molar teeth or, more frequently, their root tips, are sometimes displaced through the thin lingual plate of the mandible. This can result in local displacement nearly subperiosteal or through the mylohyoid muscle and into the submandibular space (**Fig. 5**). In this scenario, immediate stabilization of the tooth can sometimes be accomplished by placing a finger on the medial aspect along the angle of the mandible extraorally. Following stabilization, the extraction site can be widened with a small fissure bur, using caution to avoid the inferior alveolar nerve. Manual manipulation can then advance the tooth or root tip back through the extraction site for retrieval. If a root tip is especially difficult to retrieve and is at risk of dislodgement through the cortical plate, it is helpful to expose the root tip by removing the surrounding bone with a small fissure bur rather than attempting to elevate the root tip with an elevator. Elevating the root tip between the alveolus can lack control and accessibility, leading to displacement.

If the root tip finds its way through the lingual plate and below the mylohyoid muscle, a simple surgical approach can be used to dissect subperiosteal, to expose the root tip. This can be

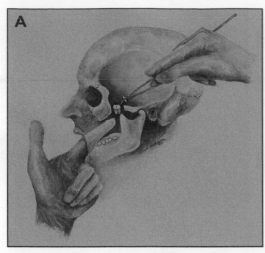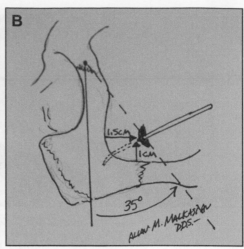

Fig. 3. (A) illustration of K wire through a supra-temporal approach while manually guiding the tooth back through an intraoral incision. Sketch and technique. (B) Demonstrates the Kirshner wire entrance point. This entrance point is made by drawing a line straight down from the zygomaticofrontal suture line, and extending another line 35° from the point of the zygomaticofrontal suture line posteriorly. Approximately l.5 cm from the distal border of the zygoma and l.0 cm above the zygomatic process of the temporal bone and anterior to this 35°angle is the entrance point made by a stab incision in the skin. This entrance point is where the Kirshner wire is introduced. (*Courtesy of* Allan Malkasian, DDS, Fresno, CA.)

accomplished by laying a full-thickness flap on the lingual border of the alveolus and dissecting subperiosteal, while maintaining digital pressure extraorally at the lingual aspect of the inferior border of the mandible (**Fig. 6**).[5] Damage to the lingual nerve is avoided if dissection is maintained subperiosteally. An extraoral incision can also be used to approach the submandibular space. One surgeon reports making a 4 mm skin incision along the submandibular region and bluntly dissecting to the lingual border of the mandible for stabilization while retrieving the object. This should be done as a last resort.[6]

A more serious, albeit rare, displacement of mandibular third molars into the lateral pharyngeal space can be daunting. When this may be perceived as a possibility, immediate CT imaging to locate and identify the tooth should be performed (**Fig. 7**). Once located, the patient should be taken to the operating room so that a secured airway via intubation can assure safety during the retrieval process. Using imaging, a small vertical incision should be made over the anticipated location of the tooth (**Fig. 8**). Then, using blunt dissection with a curved Kelly, the operator can explore the region for the tooth. Once observed, it is

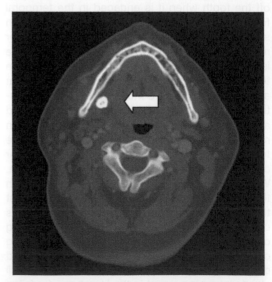

Fig. 4. Panorex of displaced mandibular third molar along the condylar neck. (*Courtesy of* Dr Dennis-Duke R. Yamashita, Montebello, CA.)

Fig. 5. Computed tomography scan illustrating displaced mandibular third molar in the submandibular space.

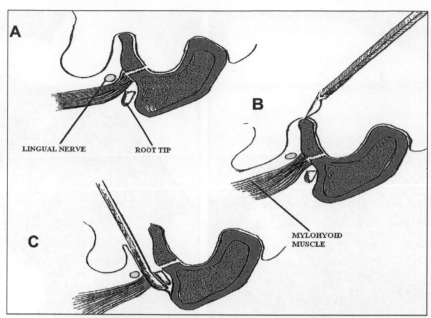

Fig. 6. Illustrating the anatomy of lingually displaced mandibular third molars. (*A*) Displaced root tip through lingual plate of the mandible as compared with lingual nerve and mylohyoid muscles. (*B*) Incision is made along the lingual border for access. (*C*) Dissection is made with periosteal elevator subperiosteal and beneath the mylohyoid muscle for access to root tip.

a matter of properly grasping the tooth with an instrument that will allow for clamping around the diameter of the tooth so as to not allow the tooth to slip away during retrieval.

Implant Misplacement

Implant misplacement is another problem that is prevented with good treatment planning and technique. Severe consequences of misdirected

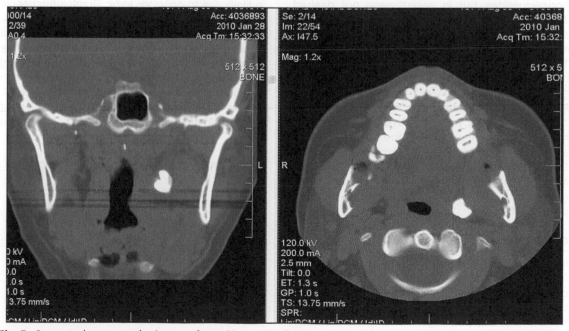

Fig. 7. Computed tomography image of mandibular third molar displaced into the lateral pharyngeal space.

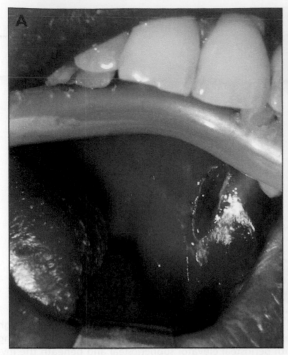
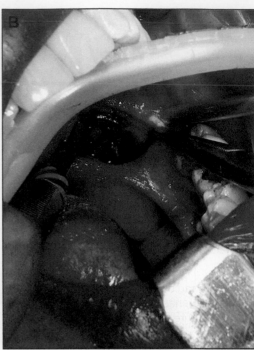

Fig. 8. (*A*) Incision over anticipated location of a displaced mandibular third molar into the lateral pharyngeal space. (*B*) Using blunt dissection to expose the displaced third molar followed by retrieval.

implants have been reported. One such consequence involved the inadvertent placement of a zygomatic implant into the cranial vault.[7] Paresthesias, anesthesia, and dysthesias can occur with cranial nerve V division 3 encroachments. Sinus encroachment can occur usually with fewer consequences but is nevertheless not desired. The use of preoperative models and imaging should be standard. Preoperative imaging, including cone beam CT, is highly recommended. The location of vital structures and available bone needs to be carefully surveyed. Proper use of guiding stents and intraoperative periapical imaging with paralleling pins will save many misdirected implants. Intraoperative occlusal assessments with guiding pins are the sine qua non of a functional and esthetic implant placement. Good control of the implants and instruments along with proper throat pack protection will greatly reduce the loss of such things down the pharynx (**Fig. 9**).

Other Displaced Objects

In addition to displaced teeth, loss of broken and faulty instrumentation during a surgical procedure can be an overwhelming complication. Instrumentation at risk for loss include injection needles, suture needles, packings, wires, plates, screws, and broken burs. In all cases, when the material

is lost, the operator is advised to immediately discontinue the procedure and make an attempt at visualizing and retrieving the material before it is further dislodged and becomes inaccessible.

Simple precautions can be used to avoid this situation. When a needle is lost during injection it is likely due to operator error. Burying the needle to the hub during a block is not advised, because it surely guarantees difficult retrieval should it break at its weakest point. Repeated use of the same needle increases the risk of breakage and should be avoided. If a needle is lost, intervention radiology-guided localization can be helpful, should local exploration fail. The insertion of a directional guide wire (ie, spinal needle) in

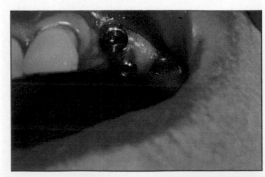

Fig. 9. Picture of poorly planned implant placement.

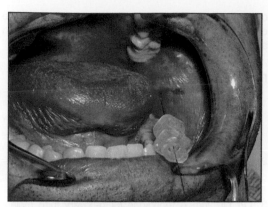

Fig. 10. Picture of needle placement along rami of mandible for reference in localizing a lost needle. Once needle is inserted, a radiograph is taken and can be used for localization.

addition to a radiograph can assist in maintaining a point of reference when exploring for the needle (**Fig. 10**). Suture needles, when lost, can also benefit from local exploration and radiographic localization. Maintaining counts, for all of the ancillary armamentarium, can be a simple precaution in avoiding this complication.

Similarly, lost burs can be avoided by the previously mentioned precautions. In addition, it is advised to use a new bur on every surgical case, as the savings of the minimal cost do not justify the repercussions of a broken bur (**Figs. 11** and **12**). Screws can also be easily lost during a procedure due to the restricted field of vision with commonly used magnification loops. Suctioning screws into the suction canister can be avoided by using small suction tips that are no bigger than the largest screw head. Unaccounted wires lost during an open reduction or osteotomy fixation with an open incision site can be avoided by cutting 1 wire at a time and confirming its removal in sequence. A postoperative panoramic image should routinely be taken following arch bar removal, as it is very easy to lose small fragments within the interproximals of the dentition.

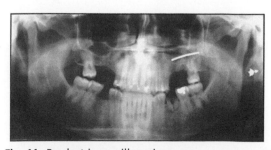

Fig. 11. Bur lost in maxillary sinus.

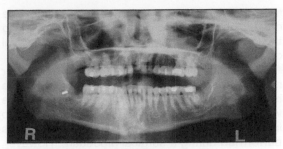

Fig. 12. Bur lost in extraction site.

The blade of an oscillating saw used during an intraoral vertical ramus osteotomy can break and get dislodged between the edges of an incomplete cut. Avoiding undue strain on the blade and overuse is advised. Retrieval of a broken blade can be accomplished by simply installing a new blade and manually rotating the blade without power within the incomplete osteotomy out of the cut (**Fig. 13**).[8] The teeth of the new blade and the broken blade should engage like the gears of the mechanical watch and allow for rotation of the displaced blade out of the bone.

If all attempts to remove a biocompatible needle, bur, or screw are a failure, it is not unreasonable to leave the material and follow up with the patient. The analogy can be made to a bullet

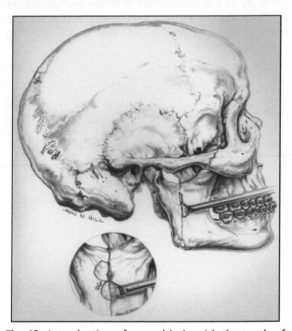

Fig. 13. Introduction of a new blade with the teeth of the blade engaged in the teeth of the broken saw blade. (*From* Tabariai E, Alexander G. An approach to retrieve a broken saw blade in an intraoral vertical ramus mandibular osteotomy. J Oral Maxillofac Surg 2008;66(11):2412–3; with permission.)

fragment left behind if inconsequential retrieval is not an option. The only disadvantage to leaving this instrumentation can result in psychological or medical–legal ramifications.

Loss of packings is different from loss of other material from the surgical armamentarium. There is more of an urgency for removal as its presence will likely result in an infection. It is difficult to imagine leaving a pack with all the safety checks performed during a surgical procedure. However, if one imagines the attempt used to achieve hemostasis during a LeFort I osteotomy down fracture one can understand how it is possible. Once plated, the packing is no longer visible to the eye during the count, which is usually performed at the end of the procedure. When found on postoperative radiography, the packing can be retrieved; however, explaining to the patient why he or she must undergo another anesthetic is not only embarrassing but can have medical–legal consequences. It is therefore advised to use absorbable homeostatic agents in case it is forgotten.

Prevention and management of displaced objects requires proper planning and surgical technique. Anticipation of untoward events and knowledge of their management is imperative. Proper informed consent should be given that includes the more common potential complications, and honesty of the occurrence of these complications is paramount for both medical–legal and ethical issues. Also, there is no shame in referring complications that are beyond the ability or the comfort of the primary surgeon to another surgeon as long as this practice is not habitual.

REFERENCES

1. Fields RT Jr, Schow SR. Aspiration and ingestion of foreign bodies in oral maxillofacial surgery: a review of the literature and report of five cases. J Oral Maxillofac Surg 1998;56:1091–8.
2. Spinnato G, Alberto PL. Complications of dentoalveolar surgery. Oral maxillofacial surgery. 2nd edition. Fonseca: Saunders Elsevier; 2009. p. 212–22.
3. Orr DL 2nd. A technique for recovery third molars from the infratemporal fossa: case report. J Oral Maxillofac Surg 1999;57:1459–61.
4. Oberman M. Accidental displacement of impacted third molars. Int J Oral Maxillofac Surg 1980;15:756–8.
5. Huang I, Wu C, Worthington P. The displaced lower third molar: a literature review and suggestions for management. J Oral Maxillofac Surg 2007;65:1186–90.
6. Yeh CJ. A simple retrieval technique for accidently displaced mandibular third molars. J Oral Maxillofac Surg 2002;60:836–7.
7. Reychler H, Olszewski R. Intracerebral penetration of a zygomatic dental implant and consequent therapeutic dilemmas: case report. Int J Oral Maxillofac Implants 2010;25(2):416–8.
8. Tabariai E, Alexander G. An approach to retrieve a broken saw blade in an intraoral vertical ramus mandibular osteotomy. J Oral Maxillofac Surg 2008; 66(11):2412–3.

Complications in Oral and Maxillofacial Surgery: Management of Hemostasis and Bleeding Disorders in Surgical Procedures

Jay P. Malmquist, DMD, FICD

KEYWORDS

- Von Willebrand disease • Hemophilia
- Coagulation factors • Platelet disorders

Oral and maxillofacial surgeons perform a wide variety of surgical procedures including the removal of teeth, various tissue biopsies, endosseous implants, and major maxillofacial surgery. One of the major complications of these various surgical techniques is uncontrolled bleeding. The best management of perioperative hemorrhage is prevention. This includes proper preoperative patient evaluation, knowledge of the various bleeding disorders, and characterization of the correct methods of management.

Hemostasis in the normal patient population involves the interaction between four different biologic systems: (1) the blood vessel wall, (2) the blood platelets, (3) the coagulation cascade, and (4) the fibrinolytic system. Under normal conditions hemostasis occurs through two independent processes: the coagulation cascade and the platelet activation pathway.[1] When the integrity of the endothelial layer of the blood vessel is compromised the initiation of the coagulation process is activated. Blood vessel constriction is the essential first stage followed by platelet adhesion and aggregation. At the site of injury the hemostatic mechanism is initiated by local activation of the surfaces and the subsequent release of tissue thromboplastin.[2] This results in the formation of fibrin. However, in oral surgery through a series of triggering steps fibrinolysis may occur

causing a breakdown of the clot. Clearly, the process is complex and requires a good level of understanding to allow the clinician to properly manage the hemostasis.

The causes of hemorrhage can be reduced to either local issues at the site of surgical intervention or inherent systemic factors. The local factors result from tissue damage at the site of surgery.[2,3] Poor surgical technique with injury to soft tissue, hard tissue, or vessels may lead to excessive bleeding. Systemic causes include the various inherited coagulation disorders, acquired coagulation abnormalities, and platelet disorders. The following discussion evaluates various causes of bleeding and identifies both local and systemic and pathways. Considerations of treatment for patients with these various disorders are discussed as to the best management options for adequate hemostasis.

SYSTEMIC FACTOR PROBLEMS

Systemic factors involving inherited coagulation disorders include von Willebrand disease, hemophilia, rare coagulation factor deficiencies, and various platelet disorders. In addition, there are acquired coagulation abnormalities and drug-induced platelet defects, which interfere with normal clot formation (**Box 1**).

Private Practice, 5415 Southwest Westgate Drive, Portland, OR 97221, USA
E-mail address: jmalmqu950@aol.com

Oral Maxillofacial Surg Clin N Am 23 (2011) 387–394
doi:10.1016/j.coms.2011.04.006
1042-3699/11/$ – see front matter © 2011 Elsevier Inc. All rights reserved.

Box 1
Common medications that affect platelet function

- American Society of Anesthesiologist (ASA)
- Nitroglycerin
- Nonsteroidal antiinflammatory drugs
- H$_2$ antagonists
- Antimicrobials
  - Penicillin
  - Ampicillin
- Propranolol
- Dipyridamole
- Sulphinpyrazone
- Clofibrate
- Tricyclic antidepressants

Von Willebrand Disease

Von Willebrand disease is the most common inherited bleeding disorder. It affects up to 1% of the population resulting in issues of surgical and nonsurgical bleeding. Increased easy bruising, epistaxis, and significant oral surgical bleeding are the most common manifestations of the disease. Von Willebrand disease results from quantitative and qualitative defects in the von Willebrand factor, an important protein in hemostasis.[4] Von Willebrand disease is divided into three different categories: type 1 is a partial deficiency of the protein factor, type 2 represents qualitative defects within the protein, and type 3 represents a severe deficiency of the total protein complex.[5]

Treatment depends on the particular type of von Willebrand disease. Most type I and some type II patients respond to desmopressin acetate, which stimulates the release of von Willebrand factor for endothelial cells. This raises the plasma level of the von Willebrand factor and factor VIII by three to five times. The half-life is approximately 8 to 12 hours, improving the primary hemostasis, and may require additional infusions. Patients who do not respond to desmopressin require pooled human plasma.[4]

Hemophilia

Hemophilia is an inherited sex-linked bleeding disorder resulting from either decreased factor VIII (hemophilia A) or factor IX (hemophilia B). The classification of hemophilia is divided into three groups: (1) severe, (2) moderate, and (3) mild. Patients with severe hemophilia have a factor level of less than 1%, moderate hemophilia represents a level of 1% to 5%, and mild hemophilia

characterizes a group of patients with factor levels between 5% and 35%. The prevalence of hemophilia is about 1 in 5000 males with up to 90% having a deficiency of factor VIII. Type B hemophilia represents only about 10% of all the diagnosed hemophilia.[6]

The classic clinical signs of a patient with a factor deficiency are bruising, muscle and joint hemorrhage, and excessive bleeding after trauma or surgical procedures. The diagnosis must be determined by specific laboratory tests. The classification often predicts the risk factors for bleeding in the specific patient.

Treatment for hemophilia is through replacement of factors VIII or IX. This is done through the use of purified plasma-derived concentrate or more recently recombinant factor concentrates. Dosage depends on the severity of the bleeding disorder.[7] Surgical procedures require preoperative doses of factor concentrations to allow for adequate control of postoperative bleeding. Occasionally, in mild cases the use of desmopressin can raise the levels of factor VIII that allow for adequate hemostasis after minor procedures.[6]

Other Congenital Factor Deficiencies

It is relatively rare to encounter other factor deficiencies. These include factors V, VII, X, and XIII. In addition, there can be deficiency of fibrinogen and prothrombin. Each of these has an occurrence rate of less than 1 in 1 million. However, when this does occur the genetic transfer is related to autosomal-recessive traits. The replacement is usually through the use of cryoprecipitate, fresh frozen plasma, recombinant factors, or various complex concentrates of the missing specific agent. One of the best ways to identify these deficiencies is to take a thorough complete medical history involving past surgical procedures.[8,9]

IATROGENIC COAGULATION ABNORMALITIES

Many patients are now being treated on a long-term basis with anticoagulation therapy using warfarin or in some cases heparin. These therapies have been researched and are now used in the prevention and management of various thrombolytic events. Thrombotic and throboembolic blockage of blood vessels are the main cause of ischemic events in the heart, lungs, and brain.[10]

Warfarin is a vitamin K antagonist, inhibiting the y-carboxylation of glutamic acid on the clotting factors. Therapeutic doses of warfarin reduce the production of functional vitamin K–dependent clotting factors by approximately 30% to 50%. Warfarin has two main functions: to cause anticoagulant activity and to provide an antithrombotic effect. Warfarin's affect is monitored by the international normalized ratio (INR; a standardization of the prothrombin time assay). The therapeutic INR range varies for most patients but is usually in the 2 to 3 range. This protects most patients from various venous or arterial thromboembolism events.[11,12] Recently, the use of hand laboratory devices allows the clinician to check the therapeutic levels of warfarin at the time of outpatient surgery. This increases the ability of the clinician to adequately evaluate the patient's risk factors for bleeding.

Heparin is a proteoglygan that functions as a cofactor of the naturally occurring anticoagulant antithrombin. Because the half-life of heparin is short (60 minutes), the therapeutic levels are maintained by intravenous bolus injections followed by monitored infusion. The therapeutic range is monitored by prolongation of the activated partial thromboplastin time. There are several different types of heparin. Low-molecular-weight heparin has a longer half-life and can be delivered subcutaneously once or twice a day. Patients on long-term therapy with heparin do not require laboratory monitoring; however, when monitoring is required a test evaluating the anit-Xa assay is used because the partial thromboplastin time is not predictably prolonged.[13]

PLATELET DISORDERS AND ABNORMALITIES

Platelet disorders can routinely be divided into two categories: defects of function or defects related to the total number of platelets. This can also include a combination of defects of the total numbers and of function. Broadly speaking, they can include the various thrombocytopenias, defects of adhesion, aggregation defects, and granular defects. In addition, there is an entire category of drug-induced defects (**Box 2**).

Throbocytopenias

The normal range for platelet levels falls within the range of 150 to 400 × 109/L however can vary for a given person into a narrower range. The platelet is routinely synthesized by the bone marrow and then destroyed by the spleen. Abnormalities generally are placed into two broad categories: those of inherited abnormalities and those of acquired abnormalities. Acquired abnormalities are relatively rare and usually represent a change in size and are associated with a specific syndrome.[14]

More common is acquired thrombocytopenia. This condition can be related to either an immune response or is of nonimmune origin. The most common immune response is thrombocytopenic

---

> **Box 2**
> **Common drugs causing thrombocytopenia**
>
> - Quinine/quinidine group
> - Heparin
> - Gold salts
> - Antimicrobials
> - Antiinflammatory drugs
> - Cardiac medications and diuretics
> - Benzodiazepines
> - Antiepileptic drugs
> - H_2 antagonists
> - Sulfonylurea drugs
> - Iodinated contrast agents
> - Retinoids
> - Antihistamines
> - Illicit drugs
> - Antidepressants
> - Miscellaneous drugs
>   - Tamoxifen
>   - Actinomycin-D
>   - Papverine

---

purpura. Often this is related to an acute infection or as a portion of a greater autoimmune syndrome.[15]

The nonimmune causes of thrombocytopenia are generally related to drug toxicity or some underlying disease state. Various chemotherapeutic agents can cause thrombocytopenia resulting in increased bleeding if the overall count drops below 50 × 109/L. The improvement of the platelet count can be accomplished by the use of platelet transfusions before surgical procedures. It is imperative that the platelets be evaluated before surgery for anyone who is being treated actively with chemotherapeutic agents.

In addition to the thrombocytopenias, there are adhesion defects, aggregation defects, and granular defects. Platelet adhesion defects result from abnormalities of the various protein complexes. There are four primary proteins involving the adhesive receptors. Genetically there can be abnormalities of any of these proteins resulting in poor platelet adhesion and associated mucosal bleeding, surgical bleeding, or easy bruisability. When this diagnosis is defined, it usually requires a platelet transfusion before a surgical procedure.[16,17]

Aggregation defects of the platelets are rare. Platelet–platelet interaction is critical to clot formation and depends on the integrity of the proteins in the integrin complex. The defect in this diagnosis is an autosomal-recessive trait caused by qualitative or quantitative problems within the protein complex. As a result of this defect there are problems of platelet aggregation resulting in bleeding and in clot retraction. This not only causes acute bleeding issues but also impacts long-term wound healing. In most cases of this genetic disorder, the signs of abnormal bleeding are diagnosed early in life and are related to bruising, epistaxis, and prolonged bleeding related to surgical procedures.

Granular defects can also impact the coagulation cascade resulting in prolonged bleeding after minor surgical procedures. Essentially, platelets contain two important storage granules: alpha granules and dense granules. Each of these granules is released after activation and is critical to the overall hemostatic mechanism. Studies have shown that both types of granules can be decreased in number and lead to prolonged bleeding. In rare instances there can be qualitative deficiencies of both granules leading to episodes of bleeding. Some have suggested that this is caused by the absence of secreted ADP.[18]

Bleeding associated with milder defects of the granules can be treated with desmopressin; however, the outcome of this therapy is difficult to predict and a trial of the desmopressin is suggested before a major procedure.

Drug-Related Platelet Defects

The most common issues with regards to platelet function are the alteration of the platelet related to ingested drugs. There are a variety of drugs both prescribed and over-the-counter medications that alter the platelet through function or through decreased numbers.

The relationship of decreased numbers of platelets and medications is not uncommon. Gold therapy, quinidine, and certain antibiotic combinations can cause marked decreased numbers of platelets. In addition, some patients who have received heparin therapy developed thrombocytopenia. This can occur in 5% to 40% who receive this type of treatment.[19]

Platelet function can be altered by several medications; however, the most common is aspirin therapy. Aspirin attenuates platelet activity through the blockage of the TxA2 release from the platelet. This is a permanent blockage and renders the platelet dysfunctional for its life. This results in aspirin therapy causing bleeding and antithrombotic activity for the life of the platelet.[20]

Several other medications can cause altered platelet function. Unlike aspirin, the nonsteroidial antiinflammatory drugs only inhibit the function of the platelet during the time that the drug is in direct contact with the platelet. Once the blood concentration is diminished there is no longer an abnormal affect on the platelet. In addition to the nonsteroidial drugs several other medications that can be obtained over the counter can cause altered function. Various H_1 antagonists, antibiotics, antidepressants, early β-blockers, and nitroglycerine have all been implicated in causing function impairment.[21]

SURGICAL TREATMENT CONSIDERATIONS IN PATIENTS WITH VARIOUS BLEEDING DISORDERS

Clearly, the most important aspect of bleeding complications is the ability to prevent a significant event from occurring. This should take into account the proposed surgical procedure and the nature of the bleeding disorder. The type of surgery, the location of the intervention, and the extent of the procedure impact how the potential problem can be avoided. Therefore, the ability to blend the issues of systemic intervention with the local interaction of the tissues impacts the overall safety and efficacy of the procedure.

Several considerations need to be addressed with regards to the surgical event. The first is the site of the surgery and ability locally to control the issues of bleeding. For instance, the removal of tooth in the anterior maxilla makes local control of that area quite easy and does not cause the clinician to manipulate the systemic issues with regards to bleeding abnormalities. However, dissection deep into the neck requires adequate safe guards to prevent hemorrhage into the neck and subsequent airway compromise. Therefore, the surgical location becomes very important in the planning stages of a procedure to prevent uncontrolled hemorrhage or hematoma formation. Such considerations as the type of local anesthesia block or infiltration may be paramount to the safe management of the patient and their systemic disorder. It may be possible to infiltrate the area with local anesthesia, obtain good local pain control, and not require the patient to undergo systemic alteration of their drug regime or various types of transfusions. Clearly, the surgical technique for the removal of a single tooth may need to be altered so that there is a minimum of trauma, reducing need for postsurgical control of the bleeding.

One of the more common questions is the influence of oral anticoagulants on oral surgical procedures and whether the particular anticoagulant needs to be altered. There are several studies that have been completed in the last 10 years stating that the discontinuance of oral anticoagulation therapy does not lead to a higher risk of postoperative bleeding.[22] It is now generally accepted

Box 3 **Recommended therapeutic range for warfarin therapy**

• Low-intensity (INR goal 2.5 with a range of 2–3)
   ○ Prophylaxis of venous thrombosis (high-risk surgery)
   ○ Treatment of venous thrombosis
   ○ Treatment of pulmonary embolism
   ○ Prevention of systemic embolism
   ○ Tissue heart valves
   ○ Acute myocardial infarction
   ○ Atrial fibrillation
• High-intensity (INR goal 3 with range of 2.5–3.5)
   ○ Most mechanical prosthetic heart valves
   ○ Prevention of recurrent myocardial infarction
 	
Data from Refs.[21,23–26]

that patients with an INR of between 2 and 4 may be treated safely without discontinuation (**Box 3**).[22]

In those patients who still have some postoperative bleeding, topical hemostatic agents are effective. More recently, dental implant therapy has been questioned as to whether it is appropriate to perform these procedures in the presence of active anticoagulation therapy. Again, the evidence does not support stopping therapy.[27] Larger, more invasive procedures, such as bone grafts, may require some alteration of the INR to ensure that there are no postsurgical bleeding complications. In addition to the use of warfarin therapy, it is also adequate to maintain low-dose aspirin therapy (100 mg/day) in the face of minor oral surgical procedures.[23]

In the past, minor oral surgical procedures in patients with hemophilia or von Willebrand disease required hospitalization and associated transfusions (**Fig. 1**). These transfusions using replacement factors carried a substantial risk of viral infection or the formation of various factor inhibitors.[28] Today, the use of recombinant non–plasma-derived products reduces this risk. One of the key agents is desmopressin treatment, which induces the release of factor VIII and von Willebrand factor. Often, these agents must be combined with local hemostatic agents or antifibrinolytic agents.[29]

Key preventive measures in patients with bleeding disorders include the following:

1. Avoid flap procedures when possible.
2. Consider techniques to minimize trauma to the area, such as limiting the number of teeth removed or the sectioning of difficult teeth.
3. Totally eliminate the associated granulation tissue in tooth sockets or the surrounding areas.
4. Consider primary closure where flaps have been elevated.
5. Use nonresorbable sutures to control the tension on the flap and eliminate the possibility of premature breakdown of the suture material.
6. Use hemostatic materials, such as the chitosan dental dressing, in the surgical site topically to reduce bleeding.
7. Use lasers or electrocautery to reduce bleeding at the time of surgical intervention.
8. Use fibrin sealants, such as Tinsel, to stabilize the fibrin clot.
9. Topical rinses, such as tranexamic acid, to inhibit fibrinolysis.
10. Use various pressure dressings to the appropriate locations of the oral cavity can be very beneficial to the control of bleeding even in the compromised patient.

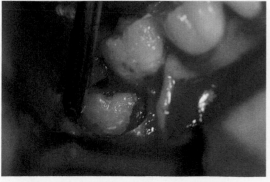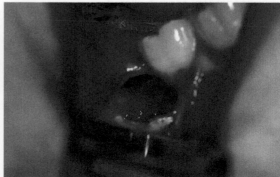

Fig. 1. Example of a minor oral surgical procedure.

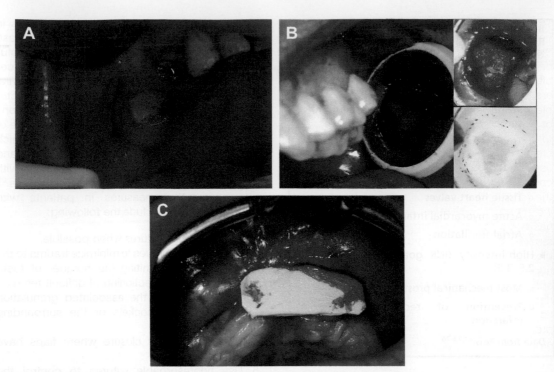

Fig. 2. (*A–C*) The use of the chitosan bandage for socket hemostasis.

11. Treat the patient early in the day, allowing for observation throughout the day for any bleeding problems.
12. The risk of significant bleeding in patients on oral anticoagulants and with a stable INR in the normal therapeutic range of 2 to 4 is extremely small and the risk of increased thrombosis in patients who are withdrawn from anticoagulants outweighs the risk of bleeding from the intraoral procedure. Oral anticoagulants should not be withdrawn from most patients who are undergoing outpatient oral surgical procedures.
13. Patients who are undergoing oral surgical procedures and who must be covered with a single dosage of antibiotics for prophylaxis against endocarditis do not need to have their anticoagulant regime altered.

THE MANAGEMENT OF POSTOPERATIVE HEMORRHAGING

Occasionally, and regardless of the techniques used, there is the postsurgical episode of bleeding requiring early intervention. This often occurs within the first 24-hour period and requires additional treatment. The most effective way to control the bleeding is to use an application of pressure to the wound area. Very often this is not well understood by the patient and even sometimes by the clinician. An adequate application of pressure to

the wound area for 30 minutes or longer very often is the only procedure needed to control the bleeding. However, in more remote cases the application of additional materials may be needed to control the oozing or frank bleeding.

Various materials have been advocated for placement into the tooth socket or wound, such as gelatin materials (Gel foam); hemostatic collagen products, such as Collatape or Helistat; and various cellulose products or even bone wax. More recently, the use of chitosan-derived hemostatic bandages for intraoral use has changed the approach to topical hemostasis (**Fig. 2**). Termed the "HemCon bandage," this chitosan bandage when topically applied intraorally can stop the excessive bleeding through a process independent of the intrinsic or extrinsic pathways of hemostasis. The negatively charged cells interact with the positively charged HemCon bandage forming an adhesive viscous clot, which seals the wound and then activates the other various coagulation pathways. This material adds an additional pathway to stopping an acute bleed and allows the clinician the ability to treat those patients who have compromised INR readings in the face of anticoagulant therapy.[30]

SUMMARY

The possibility of postoperative bleeding exists whenever a surgical procedure is undertaken.

This is further complicated when the patient is being treated with continuous oral anticoagulant therapy to decrease the risk of thromboembolism or has an inherited problem with a particular bleeding disorder. Particular treatment regimes are followed to minimize the risk of postoperative bleeding. It is now quite clear that the alteration of anticoagulant therapy is no longer necessary to decrease the incidence of postoperative bleeding after oral and maxillofacial surgery. The use of common conservative techniques in conjunction with hemostatic materials allows for the continued treatment of patients who previously were thought to be at risk for bleeding problems. It has been shown that patients who undergo oral surgery procedures have no greater risk toward bleeding than patients with normal coagulation numbers. Close collaboration with the patient and their primary physician can eliminate the need to interfere with ongoing medications for anticoagulation therapy. Safe, effective surgery and proper management of the patient can provide a predictable atmosphere for healing.

REFERENCES

1. Mann KG. Biochemistry and physiology of blood coagulation. Thromb Haemost 1999;82(2):165–74.
2. McNicol A, Israels SJ, Gerrard JM. Platelets. In: Poller L, editor. Recent advances in blood coagulation. Churchill Livingston; 1993. p. 16–80.
3. McNicol A, Gerrard JM. Platelet morphology, aggregation, and secretion. In: Lapetina EG, editor. Advances in molecular and cell biology. London: JAI Press; 1997. p. 2–28.
4. Hambleton J. Diagnosis and incidence of inherited von Willebrand disease. Curr Opin Hematol 2001; 8(5):945–51.
5. Israels LG, Israels ED. Von willenbrand factor. In: Israels LG, editor. Mechanisms in hematology. 3rd edition. Concord (MA): Core Publishing; 2002. p. 341–8.
6. Bolton-Maggs PH, Pasi KJ. Haemophilias A and B. Lancet 2003;361(9371):1801–9.
7. Gill JC. The role of genetic in inhibitor formation. Thromb Haemost 1999;82(2):500–4.
8. Peyvandi F, Mannucci PM. Rare coagulation disorders. Thromb Haemost 1999;82(4):1207–14.
9. Di Paola J, Nugent D, Young G. Current therapy for rare factor deficiencies. Haemophilia 2001;7(Suppl 1): 16–22.
10. Herman WW, Konzelman JL, Sutley SH. Current perspectives on dental patients receiving coumarin anticoagulant therapy. J Am Dent Assoc 1997;128: 327–35.
11. Israels LG, Israels ED. Vitamin K. In: Israels LG, Israels ED, editors. Mechanisms in hematology.
3rd edition. Concord (MA): Core Publishing; 2002. p. 349–54.
12. Hirsh J, Poller L. The international normalized ratio: a guide to understanding and correcting its problems. Arch Intern Med 1994;154:282–8.
13. Schafer AL. Low-molecular-weight heparin—an opportunity for home treatment of venous thrombosis. N Engl J Med 1996;334(11):724–6.
14. Drachman JG. Inherited thrombocytopenia: when a low platelet count does not mean ITP. Blood 2004;103(2):390–8.
15. Geddis AE, Kaushansky K. Inherited thrombosytopenias: toward a molecular understanding of disorders of platelet production. Curr Opin Pediatr 2004;16(1):15–22.
16. Clemetson KJ. Platelet glycoproteins and their role in diseases. Transfus Clin Biol 2001;8(30):155–62.
17. Cattaneo M. Inherited platelet-based bleeding disorders. J Thromb Haemost 2003;1(7):1628–30.
18. McNicol A, Israels SJ. Platelet dense granules: structure, function and implications for haemostasis. Thromb Res 1999;95(1):1–18.
19. Merritt JC, Bhatt DL. The efficacy and safety of perioperative antiplatelet therapy. J Thromb Thrombolysis 2002;13:97–103.
20. Antithrombotic Trialists' Collaboration. Collaborative meta-analysis of randomized trials of antiplatelet therapy for prevention of death, myocardial infarction, and stroke in high risk patients. BMJ 2002; 324:71–86.
21. Little JW, Miller CS, Henry RG, et al. Antithrombotic agents: implications in dentistry. Oral Surg Oral Med Oral Pathol Oral Radiol Endod 2002;93(5): 544–51.
22. Berine OR. Evidence to continue oral anticoagulant therapy for ambulatory oral surgery. J Oral Maxillofac Surg 2005;63:540–5.
23. Aframian DJ, Lalla RV, Peterson DE. Management of dental patients taking common hemostasis altering medications. Oral Surg Oral Med Oral Pathol Oral Radiol Endod 2007;103(Suppl):S45.e1–11.
24. Lockhart PB, Gibson J, Pond SH, et al. Dental management considerations for the patient with an acquired coagulopathy. Part 2: coagulopathies from drugs. Br Dent J 2003;195(9):495–501.
25. Carter G, Goss AN, Lloyd J, et al. Current concepts of the management of dental extraction for patients taking warfarin. Aust Dent J 2003;48(2):89–96 [quiz: 138].
26. Hirsh J, Dalen JE, Deykin D, et al. Oral anticoagulants, mechanism of action, clinical effectiveness, and optimal therapeutic range. Chest 1992; 102(Suppl 4):312S–26S.
27. Madrid C, Sanz M. What influence do anticoagulants have on oral implant therapy? A systemic review. Clin Oral Implants Res 2009;20(Suppl 4): 96–106.

28. Royer JE, Bates WS. Management of von Wille-brands's disease with desmopressin. J Oral Maxillo-fac Surg 1988;46:313–4.
29. Mannucci PM, Ruggeri ZM, Pareti FI, et al. I-deami-no-8-D-arginine vasopressin: a new pharmacolog-ical approach to the management of haemophilia and Von Willebrand's disease. Lancet 1977;1(8017): 869–72.
30. Malmquist JP, Clemens SC, Oien HJ, et al. Hemo-stasis of oral surgery wounds with the HemCon dental dressing. J Oral Maxillofac Surg 2008;66(6): 1177–83.

Dentoalveolar Nerve Injury

Thomas G. Auyong, DDS[a], Anh Le, DDS, PhD[b,c],*

KEYWORDS
- Nerve injury • Dentoalveolar • Inferior alveolar nerve
- Lingual nerve

Nerve injury associated with dentoalveolar surgery is a complication contributing to the altered sensation of the lower lip, chin, buccal gingivae, and tongue. This surgery-related sensory defect is a morbid postoperative outcome that is upsetting to the patient and should be avoided because recovery from nerve injury can be unpredictable. Several risk factors have been proposed, including advanced age, the difficulty of the operation, and the surgeon's experience, but most important, is the anatomic proximity of the third molar to the nerve canal. This article reviews the incidence of trigeminal nerve injury, presurgical risk assessment, classification, and surgical coronectomy versus conventional extraction as an approach to prevent neurosensory damage associated with dentoalveolar surgery.

INCIDENCE OF DENTOALVEOLAR NERVE INJURY

Injury to branches of the trigeminal nerve is one of the possible complications associated with the removal of third molars that markedly affect the quality of life of affected patients. Worldwide, the incidence of injury to the inferior alveolar nerve (IAN) has been reported from 0.26% to 8.4%, whereas lingual nerve (LN) deficits range from 0.1% to 22%.[1–3] In a recent prospective study at a teaching dental hospital, it was shown that, of 3595 patients with 4338 lower third molar extractions between 1998 to 2005, 0.35% developed IAN deficit, and 0.69% developed LN deficit.[2] The position of the impacted tooth, specifically the distoangular impaction, was found to increase the risk

of LN deficit significantly ($P<.001$). Another significant risk of IAN deficit is the depth of the tooth impaction ($P<.001$). Other risk factors such as sex, age, lingual flap, protection of LN with a retractor, removal of distolingual cortex, tooth sectioning, and difficulty in tooth elevation were not significantly related to IAN or LN injury. In this study, postoperative recovery from IAN and LN deficits was noted most significantly at 3 and 6 months, respectively. Almost half of the patients who sustained IAN injury had recovered by 3 months, and most of those who showed complete recovery had done so by 1 year (60%). The rate of permanent neurosensory deficit of the IAN was 0.12%. In LN deficit, the total recovery was reported in most patients (58%) within the first 6 postoperative months and in 72% patients at 2 years follow-up, and the rate of permanent neurosensory deficit was 0.16%. Results of a national survey of oral and maxillofacial surgeons reported a slightly different pattern of injuries to the IAN and LN.[4] In this report, the functional alteration rate of IAN was 1 in every 241 patients, with about 3.5% of these alterations persisting for more than a year, whereas, the lingual nerve had a functional alteration rate of 1 in every 1756 patients, with about 13% of these alterations persisted for more than a year. Based on a study of dental referral to a university-based practice setting, 52% of patients experienced some trigeminal neurosensory deficits following third molar removal.[5] Upon neurosensory evaluation, the IAN was the most commonly injured nerve (61.1%), followed by the LN (38.8%). Overall, temporary deficit in the IAN

a Department of Hospital Affairs, Ostrow School of Dentistry of the University of Southern California, 925 West 34th Street, Los Angeles, CA 90089-0641, USA
b Department of Oral and Maxillofacial Surgery, Ostrow School of Dentistry of the University of Southern California, 925 West 34th Street, Los Angeles, CA 90089-0641, USA
c Center for Craniofacial Molecular Biology, 2250 Alcazar Street, CSA 107, Los Angeles, CA 90033, USA
* Corresponding author.
E-mail address: anhle@usc.edu

Oral Maxillofacial Surg Clin N Am 23 (2011) 395–400
doi:10.1016/j.coms.2011.05.001
1042-3699/11/$ – see front matter © 2011 Published by Elsevier Inc.

injury risk ranges from 0.4% to 6 % and permanent (>6 months) injury risk is less than 1%.[6] Overall, it is believed that the close proximity of the mandibular third molar to the IAN is the primary risk factor; more specifically, it is the lack of cortical integrity of the inferior alveolar canal in relation to the mandibular third molar roots. The IAN has 4 possible positions in relation to the mandibular third molar roots: lingual, buccal, inferior, and interradicular. If there is no cortical bone between the inferior alveolar nerve and the roots (**Fig. 1**), then there is 11.8 % higher incidence of paresthesia as compared to a case with an intact cortex of the inferior alveolar canal.[7] Also, when the nerve was positioned lingually with no cortical integrity, there was a higher incidence of paresthesia. The exposure of the IAN, as observed intraoperatively, potentially incurs a higher risk for injury to the nerve than if it is not visualized.

The type and incidence of nerve damage can differ based on the technique and instrumentation used in removing third molars. The perforation of the lingual plate and the lingual bone split technique frequently used in the 1800s have been found to be associated with a higher incidence of LN damage.

RISK ASSESSMENT: ANATOMY AND IMAGING STUDIES

A major challenge for oral and maxillofacial surgeons is the inability to predict dentoalveolar surgery-related nerve injury. One contributing factor is the variable anatomic courses of both the inferior alveolar and lingual nerves. The LN passes along the mandibular ramus and lateral to the medial pterygoid muscle.[8,9] The LN's position in the pterygomandibular space makes it susceptible to injury by injection.[10] A needle directed toward the lingula will encounter the lingual nerve on its way in, because the lingual nerve is medial to the inferior alveolar nerve. Direct penetration is not the only cause of nerve damage, since adjacent

events can occur, including extraneural or intraneural hemorrhage or neurotoxic effects of local anesthetic. Its position along the mandibular ramus also makes the lingual nerve vulnerable to damage from a dentoalveolar surgical procedure even though it can actually lie either above the lingual plate or at the alveolar crest. Paralleling the inferior alveolar nerve, but lying anterior and medial to it, the LN runs below the lateral pterygoid muscle. The other vulnerable position is in the periosteum, which covers the medial wall of the third molar socket. The nerve finally enters the tongue after looping around the Wharton duct and crossing it twice.

The IAN follows the course of the inferior alveolar artery and enters the mandible at the mandibular foramen approximately 1.5 to 2 cm below the mandibular notch. The inferior alveolar nerve exits the mandible at the mental foramen commonly located near the apex of the second mandibular premolar, but it can also be anterior or posterior to this position. The IAN, at this point now called the mental nerve, supplies sensation to the skin of the chin and the lower lip. Impacted lower third molars can be juxtaposed to the course of the IAN in the posterior mandible and therefore comprise the primary surgical challenge and risk of injury to this nerve.

Imaging of the location of the inferior alveolar nerve is obviously the best way to avoid complications. Imaging techniques have their advantages and disadvantages, risks and benefits. The most common method of imaging is the panoramic radiograph. The advantage of this image is the ease of obtaining an image, cost effectiveness, and relatively low radiation exposure. The disadvantages of this image are the lack of 3-dimensional spatial relationships, lack of definitive details in the image, and magnification of the image, which can be variable.

Several features on panoramic radiographs have been described to guide the prediction of the proximity of the tooth to the IAN based on the subtle loss of cortical integrity, including: interruption of the

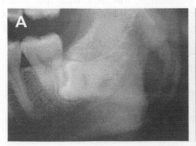 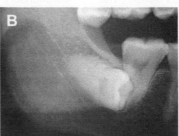 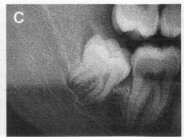

Fig. 1. Radiographs of relationship of inferior alveolar nerve and lower third molars showing interruption of the white cortical outline (*A–C*), diversion of the mandibular canal (*A*), and darkening of roots (*C*).

white line of the inferior alveolar canal, darkening of the roots, diversion of the canal, narrowing of the canal, narrowing of the roots, and deflection of the roots. Of these, only 3 features are accurate in predicting inferior alveolar nerve exposure,[6] which include the interruption of the white line, darkening of the roots, and deviation of the mandibular canal (see **Fig. 1**). The most significant factor to predict nerve exposure is the presence of the darkening outline around the root apexes.

Recently, another addition to imaging has been the cone beam computed tomography (CBCT). Although cost and radiation exposure are disadvantages, CBCT not only can detect the presence of IAN exposure, but also the degree of exposure. It has been found that if the exposure is greater than 3 mm (as seen on 3 tomographic sections), there is a 20% increase in risk of IAN damage.[7] Since the lingual position of the mandibular canal is significantly associated with IAN injury, CBCT can elucidate the 3-dimensional relationship of the third molar root and allow a buccolingual visualization of the canal to identify cases in which a lingually placed IAN is at risk during surgery.

CLASSIFICATION OF NERVE INJURY

There are several mechanisms to classify nerve injuries (**Table 1**). In most systems, the classification is based on clinical symptoms or microanatomy or gross appearance of the nerve damage. These classifications emphasize on the severity of the injury and the potential for recovery. The oldest and most commonly referred system is Seddon's classification proposed in 1943 categorized as neuropraxia, axonotmesis, and neurotmesis.[11] Neuropraxia is defined as a conduction block without axonal damage. The anatomic continuity of both the sheath and the axon is maintained. The nonfunctioning axon is attributed to focal demyelination. This is usually from a mild trauma (bruising or concussion) and resolves within hours to a few months. Axonotmesis is a result of moderate trauma (stretching or crushing), which is characterized by nerve fiber degeneration distal to the point of injury (Wallerian degeneration). This type of injury can recover, but the recovery can be variable and partial. Neurotmesis is a severe injury characterized by the direct transection of the nerve and a resulting distal degeneration. Recovery cannot spontaneously occur.

Sunderland in 1951 sought to improve nerve injury classification based on the level of anatomic injury. There were 5 levels or degrees of nerve injury. Each higher level would include the degree of injury from the preceding level. Degree 1 is an intact nerve with local conduction block. There can be some demyelinization. Recovery is expected to be complete in 2 to 3 weeks.[12] This would correspond to Seddon's neuropraxia. Seddon's axonotmesis would encompass degree 2 through 4 in Sunderland's classification. Degree 2 is defined as injury to the axon only. Wallerian

Table 1
Classification systems and characteristics of sensory nerve injuries

Seddon	Sunderland	Histologic Observation	Recovery	Prognosis
Neuropraxia	1	Nerve trunk and axon continuity Demyelination	Complete in days to weeks	Excellent
Axonotmesis	2	Axon disruption involving endoneurium or/and perineurium	Complete in 3–6 months	Good to excellent
	3	Demyelination Progressively more axon damage	Incomplete after 3–6 months	Fair to good
Neurotmesis	4	Nerve trunk disruption involving endoneurium, perineurium and epineurium Demyelination	Incomplete after 3–6 months	None to poor
	5	Partial or complete transection	No sensation or incomplete after 3–6 months	None to poor

degeneration does occur; however, the nerve regenerates by following the intact endoneurial tubule. Recovery occurs at a rate of 1mm/d. Degree 3 injury has damage to the endoneurium. A torn endoneurial tube slows healing, and recovery can be incomplete. Degree 4 injury now has damage to the perineurium. The loss of the fascicular structure can lead to the formation of neuroma-in-continuity. The epinerium is intact, but the fascicles are disorganized, either narrowed or expanded.[12] The failure to reach the peripheral target can result in pain. Degree 5 is a total transection and loss of continuity. There is no hope of recovery from this injury without surgical repositioning of the nerve ends. The proximal and distal ends form the amputation or stump neuroma. This disorganized structure is made up of microsprouts and unoriented fascicles.[9] This last level corresponds to Seddon's neurotmesis.

Another classification system is based upon symptoms. This system has 3 categories and is discussed by LaBlanc.[11] The categories are: anesthesia (complete absence of any stimulus detection or perception); paresthesia (appropriate, but abnormal stimulus detection or perception); and dysesthesia (inappropriately abnormal stimulus detection or perception). Paresthesia includes hypoesthesia (decreased sensation), hyperesthesia (increased sensation), hypoalgesia (decreased appropriate pain sensation), and hyperalgesia (increased appropriate pain sensation). Dysesthesia has a painful response to inappropriate stimuli such as allodynia, which is a sharp pain provoked by a light touch. Although this classification system is more clinical in its orientation, it does not explain the origin of the injury. Some of the causes are not necessarily the disruption of the axons.

NERVE DEGENERATION AND REGENERATION

Nerve injury sets in motion many mechanisms of degeneration and then regeneration.[9] The cells involved are the neuron, the macrophage, the Schwann cell, and the fibroblast. For neurapraxic injuries, segmental demyelinization occurs. Recovery is just a matter of remyelination, which can occur in a few hours or a few months. For more severe injuries, the axons will swell, and myelin will break down into fat droplets. As this Wallerian degeneration occurs, the damage progresses proximally and distally from the injury site. The macrophage is involved in the phagocytosis of the neural fat and cellular debris. The proximal severed stump seals over. The distal stump undergoes further Wallerian degeneration and within 6 to 8 weeks becomes only endoneurial tubes lined by Schwann cells (bands of Bungner). The Schwann cells are then activated. The Schwann cell supports the neuron by surrounding the axon with an extracellular matrix called the basal lamina or basement membrane. These Schwann cells proliferate and begin producing nerve growth factor (NGF) and other neurotrophic factors that will support axonal regeneration once the sprouts reach the distal stump. Fibroblasts will then surround the regenerating nerves to produce perineurium and aid in the formation of new fascicles. Fibroblasts can also cause excess scarring, which leads to neuroma formation (neuroma-in-continuity or stump neuroma). If the axon is unable to capture the distal stump, Schwann cells will decline, and the bands of Bungner will be infiltrated with vascular cells and fibroblasts.

Nerve regeneration will involve all 5 components of an injured nerve, the neuron, the proximal stump (nerve segment from neuron to injury), site of injury, the distal stump (nerve segment from injury to end organ), and the end organ. Repair mechanisms include remyelination, collateral sprouting from undamaged collateral axons, and regeneration from injury site. Collateral sprouting is a main mechanism in smaller injuries where only 20% to 30% of the axons are injured.[12] Regeneration from the injury site is more predominant in more severe damage, where 90% of the axons are involved. Schwann cells play an important role in assisting the sprouting axons and help attract the axon down the endoneural tube. Axonal regeneration from collateral sprouts depends upon the sprouts entering the endoneurial tubes of the distal stump. This regeneration down the endoneurial tube is estimated at 1–2 mm/d or 1 in/mo. If one supposes that the inferior alveolar nerve is 20 cm long, then nerve regeneration could take place by 3.5 to 6.6 months.[13] Again, this is a theoretic supposition, and it also must be pointed out that reaching the target organ does not necessarily mean restoration of function. Once the axon has reached the target organ, there needs to be recovery of the receptor. Another factor in regeneration of a trigeminal nerve is the survival of ganglionic neurons. Injury to a peripheral branch of the trigeminal nerve will cause to the loss of ganglionic neurons. Rath estimated a 25% and 47% reduction in trigeminal ganglionic cells with transaction of the IAN and mental nerve, respectively.[14] Zuniga furthermore defined 8 requirements for ideal peripheral sensory nerve regeneration,[13] which include: survival of ganglionic cells, axonal sprouting from proximal stump, Schwann cell proliferation, endothelial tube preservation, sprout contact with endothelial tube, downgrowth of sprouts through tube, receptor reinnervation, and fiber and receptor maturation.

CLINICAL ASSESSMENT OF NERVE INJURY

Clinical assessment of nerve injury is done not only at initial presentation, but also periodically to assess and monitor the recovery of the nerve injury. The initial assessment might also give some insight as to the type and prognosis of recovery. There have been several methods for sensory nerve assessment. Zuniga and Essick offered the most comprehensive method.[15] Steunenberg and Pogrel also detailed a similar assessment method.[16] Both of these methods assessed: pain, temperature, pressure, light touch, direction sense, and 2- point discrimination. Unfortunately, these methods are also detailed and time-consuming, making them difficult to implement on a routine clinical basis. Specialized instruments such as Von Freys hairs and Semmes-Weinstein monofilaments are needed. Several authors (Meyer and Rath,[17] Bagheri[18]) proposed the British Medical Research Council Scale (MRC) as modified by Mackinnon and Dellon to assess peripheral hand injuries.[19] This particular scaling method involved scores of S0 (no recovery) to S4 (total recovery). The simplicity of using the modified MRC scale is that it makes only 3 assessments: pain (deep and superficial), touch, and 2-point discrimination. All of these tests can be easily done with a cotton plier. An assessment of the status of the sensory nerve can be done in a relatively short time in everyday clinical setting. Coupled with a few pointed subjective questions, a concise clinical status of the nerve can be reached. The modified MRC Scale (**Table 2**) is defined as follows:

> S0 no recovery
> S1 recovery of deep cutaneous pain
> S1+ recovery of superficial pain
> S2 same as S1+ with addition of some touch sensation
> S2+ same as S2 but with hyperesthesia
> S3 same as S2 but without hyperesthesia and with 2-point discrimination greater than 15 mm,
> S3+ same as S3 with good localization of stimulus and 2-point discrimination of about 7 to 15 mm
> S4 complete recovery (2-point discrimination is now 2 to 6 mm).[17,18]

Under this system, anything graded S3 or higher is considered useful sensory recovery. For the lower lip any 2-point discrimination greater than 15 is considered abnormal with normal being less than about 8 mm. For the tongue, normal 2-point discrimination would be 5 mm for the dorsum and 1 to 2 mm for the tip.[16] LN deficit commonly presents with numbness of the ipsilateral anterior two-thirds of the tongue and taste disturbance.

Table 2
Medical Research Council scale for sensory nerve evaluation

Grade	Description
S0	No sensation
S1	Deep cutaneous pain in autonomous zone
S2	Some superficial pain and touch
S2+	Superficial pain and touch plus hyperesthesia
S3	Superficial pain and touch without hyperesthesia; static 2-point discrimination >15 mm
S3+	Same as S3 with good stimulus localization and static 2-point discrimination of 7–15 mm
S4	Same as S3 and static 2-point discrimination of 2–6 mm

Data from Birch R, Bonney G, Wynn-Parry CB. Surgical disorders of the peripheral nerves. Philadelphia: Churchill Livingstone; 1998. p. 405–14.

CORONECTOMY VERSUS EXTRACTION

Coronectomy is an alternative procedure to the complete extraction of the third molar tooth. The method involves the sectioning and removal of the crown of an impacted mandibular third molar while leaving the root undisturbed, thereby avoiding direct or indirect damage to the juxtaposed nerve. Although coronectomy was first described by B. O'Riordan at a meeting of the British Association of Oral Maxillofacial Surgeons in June 1997, the technique has yet to gain popularity because of surgeons' concerns about the short- and long-term outcomes as well as associated complications.

In a randomized study of 128 patients who required operations on mandibular third molars and had radiological evidence of proximity of the third molar to the IAN canal, 19% of nerve injuries were reported following standard extraction versus none after successful coronectomy, and 8% after failed coronectomy.[20] The incidence of dry socket and infection was similar in all the three groups. A similar study using a randomized controlled trial of 231 patients with specific radiographic signs of close proximity of wisdom teeth roots to the IAN who underwent surgery for 349 lower wisdom teeth (171 coronectomies, 178 controls), reported fewer complications in terms of neurosensory deficit, and much lower incidence of pain and dry socket in the coronectomy group as compared to the extraction group.[21] Likewise, there were no statistical differences in infection rate between the 2 groups. In a small number of coronectomy cases, the migration of retained roots has been reported with uneventful outcomes.

Since surgical management of neurosensory disturbances, specifically microvascular nerve repair, can be quite challenging and comes with variable outcomes, an alternative approach to conventional surgical extraction, such as coronectomy—if proven to be safe—could be an acceptable choice to minimize neurosensory disturbance associated with removal of wisdom teeth with high risk of nerve damage.

REFERENCES

1. Gulicher D, Gerlach KL. Sensory impairment of the lingual and inferior alveolar nerves following removal of impacted mandibular third molars. Int J Oral Maxillofac Surg 2001;30:306–12.

2. Cheung LK, Leung YY, Chow LK, et al. Incidence of neurosensory deficits and recovery after lower third molar surgery: a prospective clinical study of 4338 cases. Int J Oral Maxillofac Surg 2010;39:320–6.

3. Jerjes W, Upile T, Shah P, et al. Risk factors associated with injury to the inferior alveolar and lingual nerves following third molar surgery—revisited. Oral Surg Oral Med Oral Pathol Oral Radiol Endod 2010;109:335–45.

4. Alling CC. Dysesthesia of the lingual and inferior alveolar nerves following third molar surgery. J Oral Maxillofac Surg 1986;44:454–7.

5. Tay AB, Zuniga ZR. Clinical characteristics of trigeminal nerve injury referrals to a university centre. Int J Oral Maxillofac Surg 2007;36:922–7.

6. Park W, Choi JW, Kim JY, et al. Cortical integrity of the inferior alveolar canal as a predictor of paresthesia after third molar extraction. JADA 2010;141(3):271–8.

7. Ghaeminia H, Meijer GH, Soehardi A, et al. Position of the impacted third molar in relation to the mandibular canal. Diagnostic accuracy of cone beam computed tomography compared with panoramic radiography. Int J Oral Maxillofac Surg 2009;38:964–71.

8. Norton N. Netter's head and neck anatomy for dentistry. Philadelphia: Saunders; 2007.

9. DeBrul E. Sicher's oral anatomy. St Louis (MO): C V Mosby Company; 1980.

10. Morris C, Rasmussen J, Throckmorton G, et al. The anatomic basis of lingual nerve trauma associated with inferior alveolar block injection. J Oral Maxillofac Surg 2010;68:2833–6.

11. LaBlanc J. Classification of nerve injuries. Oral Maxillofac Surg Clin North Am 1992;4:285–95.

12. Campbell W. Evaluation and management of peripheral nerve injury. Clin Neurophysiol 2008;119: 1951–65.

13. Zuniga JR. Normal response to nerve injury. Oral Maxillofac Surg Clin North Am 1992;4:323–37.

14. Rath E. Peripheral neurotrauma-induced sensory neuropathy. Oral Maxillofac Surg Clin North Am 2001;13:223–35.

15. Zuniga J, Essick G. A contemporary approach to the clinical evaluation of trigeminal nerve injuries. Oral Maxillofac Surg Clin North Am 1992;4:353–67.

16. Steunenber A, Pogrel MA. Nerve injury: a protocol for neurological evaluation and patient care. Presented at 70th Annual Meeting of the American Association of Oral and maxillofacial Surgeon and the AAOMS Mutual Insurance Company Risk Retention Groups Risk Management Seminar. Boston (MA), September 29 to October 3, 1988.

17. Meyer R, Rath E. Sensory rehabilitation after nerve injury or nerve repair. Oral Maxillofac Surg Clin North Am 2001;13:365–76.

18. Baheri S, Meyer R, Khan H, et al. Microsurgical repair of peripheral trigeminal nerve injuries from maxillofacial trauma. J Oral Maxillofac Surg 2009; 67:1791–9.

19. Poort L, vanNeck J, van der Wal K. Sensory testing of inferior alveolar nerve injuries: a review of methods used in prospective studies. J Oral Maxillofac Surg 2009;67:292–300.

20. Rentona T, Hankinsb M, Sproatec C, et al. A randomised controlled clinical trial to compare the incidence of injury to the inferior alveolar nerve as a result of coronectomy and removal of mandibular third molars. Br J Oral Maxillofac Surg 2005; 43:7–12.

21. Leung YY, Cheung LK. Safety of coronectomy versus excision of wisdom teeth: a randomized controlled trial. Oral Surg Oral Med Oral Pathol Oral Radiol Endod 2009;108:821–7.

Alveolar Osteitis and Osteomyelitis of the Jaws

Peter A. Krakowiak, DMD, FRCD(C)[a,b,c,*]

KEYWORDS
- Osteomyelitis • Delayed healing • Marrow infection
- *Actinomyces* • Dry socket • Immune compromised

OVERVIEW

Postoperative bone healing after oral surgical procedures occurs uneventfully in most cases because of exceptional vascularity of head and neck structures when compared with other anatomic sites. However, in certain patients, the normal process of osseous healing can be delayed and, in some cases, often because of multiple co-existing factors, the sites can become infected, with extension of the infection into medullary bone. This process is termed osteomyelitis. The exact definition of osteomyelitis is inflammation of the osseous medulla. The term osteitis reflects a more superficial inflammation of the cortex of the bone. Most often, infections of the medulla also involve the cortex by the pathways of haversian systems and often affect the overlying periosteum. Hence the term osteomyelitis is more commonly used to describe alveolar and basal bone infections. The infectious process in the marrow space of bones has been well documented in early man. The oldest known case of mandibular osteomyelitis dates back to the Pleistocene epoch about 1.6 million years ago and fossil findings in the jaw of a 12-year-old *Homo erectus* skeleton found in Kenya. Since the discovery of bacteria and the advancement in antimicrobial therapy, there has been a significant decrease in the incidence with improved outcomes in the care of these infectious conditions.[1,2] Over the years, multiple classification schemes have been proposed,[1–6] but most current literature on the topic suggest wisely using a simplified classification system based on clinical course time lines and appearance of the disease.[3] This simplified classification scheme is used in discussing the pathogenesis, diagnosis, and therapy for these conditions. Imaging techniques, including the new positron emission tomography/computed tomography (PET/CT) fusion techniques, are addressed. Pathogenesis, microbiology, and surgical and medical therapies are outlined. This article specifically addresses osteomyelitis cases related to patients with no documented history of radiation or bisphosphonate exposure and in whom the principal factor in the development of the condition is infection by pyogenic microorganisms.[3] The other subsets of infectious osseous pathosis are discussed by Leon A. Assael; and Sinha and colleagues specifically elsewhere in this issue.

DENTOALVEOLAR SURGICAL WOUND HEALING

Normal wound healing is aimed at restoring the site to the preinjury state. It is often a sequential process that starts at the time of injury and is based on cellular level messing that induces homeostatic, inflammatory, angiogenic, inductive, and mitogenic changes in local cell populations as well as circulating pluripotent cell recruitment and differentiation. Site regeneration involves both metabolic and catabolic changes, which are

The author has nothing to disclose.

[a] Oral and Maxillofacial Surgery, Herman Ostrow School of Dentistry, University of Southern California, 925 West 34th Street, Room Den 146, Los Angeles, CA 90089, USA
[b] Private Practice, 265 San Jacinto River Road, Suite 101, Lake Elsinore, CA 92587, USA
[c] Private Practice, 5256 South Mission Road Suite, Bonsall, CA 92003, USA
* Lakeshore Oral and Maxillofacial Surgery, 265 San Jacinto River Road, Suite 101 Lake Elsinore, CA 92530.
E-mail address: pkoms@sbcglobal.net

Oral Maxillofacial Surg Clin N Am 23 (2011) 401–413
doi:10.1016/j.coms.2011.04.005
1042-3699/11/$ – see front matter © 2011 Elsevier Inc. All rights reserved.

influenced by local and host factors including vascularity and oxygen supply. Hypoxia decreases normal antimicrobial activity of granulocytes by as much as 50%.[7] Bacterial virulence is also a significant factor in the development of early or late wound infections.[2,3,8] Finally, host vascular and immune factors and current immune status have been shown to affect the incidence of head and neck delayed healing and wound infections.[1,8–10]

ALVEOLAR OSTEITIS (DRY SOCKET)
Incidence

One of the best known and most referred to complications of dental extraction in the general public is alveolar osteitis (AO) better known as the dry socket. It is a common postoperative complication that occurs in less than 5% of patients undergoing tooth extraction.[11–17] The research, despite high incidence of this condition, is poorly structured with rates of incidence ranging broadly from 0.5% to 37.5%.[18,19] Third molar surgery carries the highest incidence of AO occurrence. Maxillary AO is very rare and is often misdiagnosed as normal postoperative discomfort. It is widely thought that this misdiagnosis is due to higher maxillary bone vascularity because of more circumferential sources of supply over the central endosseuous mandibular pattern. The best description of the condition is premature fibrinolysis of the clot, which may result in local and radiating pain, halitosis, and abdominal discomfort.[20,21]

Cause of AO

Despite the long-term awareness of the condition, the cause of AO is still not fully understood, but it has been widely noted that premature fibrinolytic breakdown of the initial platelet clot in the extraction site exposes the underlying and tooth socket bone (**Fig. 1**). Breakdown of the clot occurs as a result of plasminogen pathway activation whereby an activator substance is triggered by either physiologic or nonphysiologic mediators (including bacterial enzymes). Specific factors are debated and poorly understood, but all of them have some promoter effect on clot lysis, which leads to fibrinolysis.[22,23] It has been postulated that bacteria is limited to the surface of the bone and does not produce a true medullary bone infection.[3,6,22] Hence at present, AO is not categorized as a true infectious process of the bone.

Symptoms

The cardinal symptom of AO is pain that originates in the jaw and radiates either from the ear to temple and/or runs in the lower jaw along the

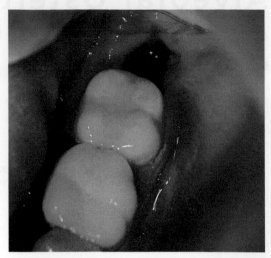

Fig. 1. Typical clinical presentation of extraction site devoid of blood clot.

trigeminal nerve distribution affecting all distal teeth and bone.[14,16,17] Other reported symptoms include low-grade fever,[20,21] halitosis,[21] exposed bone, and regional lymphadenopathy.[20,21,24]

Onset

Most patients diagnosed with AO have reported onset of symptoms after 3 to 5 days after the surgical procedure.[20,24,25] However, continued localized painful symptoms from the day of surgery are also possible. AO-like symptoms that become evident after 1 week from the surgery are not consistent with AO[11] time lines and therefore should be considered to be stemming from another process, which may include either food debris impaction or acute osteomyelitis.

Risk Cofactors in AO

The increased risk factors for development of AO have been well identified and documented in many studies and include preexisting infection, poor oral hygiene, partial impaction of tooth, periodontal disease, lack of operator experience, oral contraceptive use, tobacco use, and increased age.[16,24–27] Other factors are flap design, vasoconstrictor use, aggressiveness of site manipulation, saliva exposure, the patient's age, and the level of systemic health of patient, although their role has not been clearly demonstrated.[14,16,28]

Treatment of AO

No significant changes in the management of the condition have occurred in the past few decades. The main focus of the current therapeutic approach for AO is to maintain patient comfort for the initial healing period after surgical intervention until the normal healing process can occur. Therapy includes the application of topical analgesics and antimicrobial agents.[28]

The medications are usually applied on a carrier vehicle such as iodoform gauze, collagen, or gelatin sponge (**Fig. 2**). Many combinations exist for the treatment medication formulation, but the majority includes substances that contain eugenol with other additives such as benzocaine, guaiacol, balsam of Peru, chlorobutanol and iodoform, and others. The site is usually irrigated to remove any foreign debris and evaluated for any loose fragments of bone. Local anesthesia may be used for patient comfort but is usually not necessary. Limited manipulation of tissue is recommended. The dressing on the carrier is then applied into the site and packed to rest at the level of or slightly below the crest of the socket walls (**Fig. 3**). The drawback to placement of these carrier-based medications is that it retards some of the healing process because all dressings are foreign bodies.[28] The patient usually requires multiple dressing changes, and the exact number of changes is always dictated by the patient's relative comfort.

Premade dressings and carrier medications, such as Alvogyl (Septodont Inc Wilmington, DE, USA), that are marketed as place and dissolve dressings have been shown to produce delayed healing.[29,30] Moreover, any retained dressing can become a nidus for late infection and should be removed after 2 to 3 days in place and either discarded or replaced with a new dressing. Radiolabeled dressings, such as Dressol-X (Rainbow Specialty & Health Products Inc, Niagara Falls, NY, USA), are superior to regular iodoform dressings because they allow for easy identification if retained and overgrown by tissues.

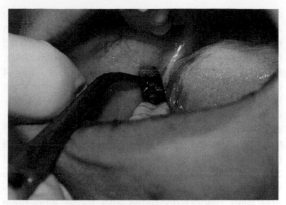

Fig. 3. Iodoform dressing being placed into third molar site using pick ups.

Patients can be prescribed additional analgesics and placed on gentle saline or 0.12% chlorhexidine rinses.[31] Moist warm heat compresses are helpful in increasing circulation and comfort in the area. Multiple agents including parahydroxybenzoic acid, polylactic acid, corticosteroids, 9-aminocrinide, and tranexamic acid have been used but have not been scientifically shown to be useful in the treatment or prevention of AO.[14,22]

AO SYNOPSIS

Although the incidence of AO is very high, especially in third molar extractions, it is a self-limiting concern, which benefits most from a few 1- to 2-day local topical treatments with eugenol-based compounds on a nonresorbable carrier. Patients who have identifiable risk factors should optimized medical therapy and appropriately counseled regarding their risks. At the same time, the practitioners should be able to differentiate between normal postoperative pain, which tends to improve after the initial 24 to 48 hours, and the increasing symptoms of AO, which become more pronounced after the 72-hour mark. In all cases, frank reassurance and prompt management of this common condition is paramount to the practitioner's ability to provide the necessary care for the patient with AO.

OSTEOMYELITIS OF THE JAW

Most osteomyelitis in long bones arise from either local extension or hematogenous spread, but in maxillofacial skeleton, the spread is mostly by local extension from skin, oral cavity, or paranasal sinuses.[1,32,33] It is a relatively uncommon complication in patients undergoing extraction with normal immune function status because of the perceived excellent vascularity in this region of the body.[1,3,6,33,34] Highest rates of osteomyelitis

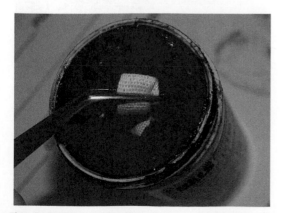

Fig. 2. Topical medication being applied to nonresorbable iodoform gauze.

are noted in patients with vascular insufficiency and immune dysfunction as well as in those with bone metabolic abnormalities. These (metabolic bone) conditions include diabetes, fibrous dysplasia, florid osseous dysplasia, osteopetrosis, Paget disease, sickle cell anemia, osseous malignancies leukemia, agranulocytosis, systemic steroids, intravenous drug use, renal and hepatic failure, and human immunodeficiency virus infection.[1,3,6] Patients who take immunosuppressive agents, are malnourished, and consume significant amounts of alcohol[3,9] are also at a higher risk. Finally, patients who have received or are receiving osteochemotherapy with bisphosphonates and those who have undergone radiation therapy are a separate and highly risk-prone segment of patients who can develop maxillomandibular osteomyelitis. These 2 specific conditions are discussed elsewhere in this issue but need to be included in the list of contributing factors. However, 17% of patients who develop osteomyelitis have no identifiable underlying predisposing factors.[35]

CLASSIFICATION SCHEMES

The classification schemes for evaluating and treating AO have been based on clinical and radiographic findings, cause, pathogenesis, and associated anatomy. However, there is no 1 set standard. The most simplistic way to consider the condition is based on an arbitrary time line of 1 month and is considered to be either acute or chronic condition. The modifier for the picture can also include a suppurative attribute. Because the suppurative form is more aggressive and often it is hard to differentiate the chronic nonsuppurative entities from various fibro-osseous ones including clinically overlapping diffuse sclerosing osteomyelitis (DSO) or periostistis ossificans (PO) or Garré osteomyelitis lesions, the more suppurative variant is discussed in more depth in this article. It is also more related to acute complications of surgical therapy, which is the focus of this article. The chronic variant of osteomyelitis is also associated with synovitis acne pustulosis hyperostosis osteitis (SAPHO) syndrome, which is characteristic for synovitis, acne, pustulosis, hyperostosis, and osteitis and may be linked to HLA-B13 and HLA-B27–related autoimmune conditions.[32]

ACUTE OSTEOMYELITIS

Within this category, the patient may experience quite a range of symptoms and varied presentations. Most cases have significant pain in the jawbones, swelling, trismus, purulent drainage, and febrile episodes with potential hypoesthesias

in more than 50% of the cases.[1,3,6] Additional clinical signs include lymphadenopathy, fistulous tracts, exposed bone, and sequestra formations (**Figs. 4** and **5**). Patients may report malaise and fatigue. Normal to slightly elevated leukocyte count is noted in most cases, but about one-third of the patients may have significantly increased leukocyte counts of more than 15,000.[6] Additional laboratory values of interest are erythrocyte sedimentation rate and C-reactive protein values, which may also be elevated. C-reactive protein values can be used to follow the resolution of infection and progress of therapy.[6,32,36] Patients who do not show significant symptoms during the acute phase and do not receive adequate therapy are considered to have subacute condition and most often progress to the chronic phase of the disease.[1,3,6,8]

CHRONIC OSTEOMYELITIS (SUPPURATIVE)

Chronic osteomyelitis occurs in patients in whom either a host resistance or a therapeutic failure occurs allowing the infectious process to continue past the 30-day mark. The symptoms and clinical presentation may be less severe than those of an acute form, but most patients still present with jaw pain, swelling, and suppuration.[6] Usually, the bone undergoes sequestra formation and demonstrates significant changes radiographically. With

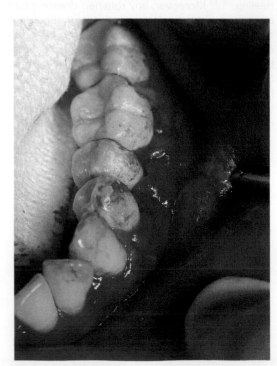

Fig. 4. Gingival edema and mobile dentition in the area of affected by osteomyelitis.

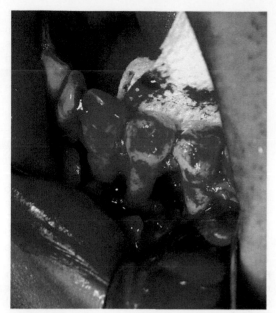

Fig. 5. After elevation of a full thickness flap extensive bone loss and necrosis is evident.

a severe degree of progression, there is a potential for pathologic fractures and formation of extraoral fistulae. The lower-grade processes tend to progress into the sclerosis variants on either DSO (medullary) or PO discussed as nonsuppurative variants.

CHRONIC OSTEOMYELITIS (NONSUPPURATIVE)

This form of medullary marrow infection is thought to be caused by overgrowth of *Actinomyces* and *Eikenella corrodens*.[3,32] It usually has milder symptoms and may be free of other clinical signs and symptoms with the exception of radiographic findings. In most cases, the disease is diagnosed several years into the disease process.[32] The lesions are often mistaken for fibro-osseous lesions and are difficult to definitively diagnose without biopsy and cultures.

OTHER RELATED CONDITIONS

PO, also known as Garré osteomyelitis, is named after Carl Garré, although he did not describe this specific condition in any of his late eighteenth century works. PO is characterized by deposition of immature bone layers over the existing cortical contour. Onion skin radiographic appearance of this expansile proliferative condition is classical but not pathognomonic because malignancy of bone may have similar appearance. No symptoms are evident in these cases.[6,32]

NEURALGIA-INDUCING CAVITATIONAL OSTEONECROSIS

Neuralgia-inducing cavitational osteonecrosis is a condition described by Dr Boquot who assigned osseous osteomyelitis–like changes to patients with atypical facial pain and neuralgia.[32] Patients were then subjected to experimental protocols including curettage and bone graft protocols that were aimed at reducing symptoms. Since gaining some attention in the early 1990s, the condition has not been more scientifically defined in the peer-reviewed literature, and the practitioners of this methodology have been involved in extended legal battles, disciplinary actions, and class action suits. Limited literature supports the existence of this condition, and most is the work of its inventors and proponents. There are many who have discredited the existence and validity of the treatments proposed for this obscure and controversial pathosis.[32,37,38]

DIAGNOSTIC IMAGING

The increasing availability of 3-dimensional imaging, magnetic resonance imaging (MRI), scintigraphy, and, now, PET/CT imaging has made it much easier to precisely delineate the extent of the disease process in a timely manner. The newest imaging modalities, such as scintigraphy and PET scan, are able to highlight biological as well as anatomic activity and may be coupled with navigational approaches to virtual surgical therapy and interventions.[6,39]

Conventional Radiography

Albeit the standard for many decades, the role of this modality is limited in detection of and therapy for osteomyelitis because it only shows changes after extensive bone abnormality has been present for prolonged periods.[40] However, it is readily available and exposes patients to minimal radiation. Panoramic projection is most useful in most maxillofacial cases (**Fig. 6**).

CT

The addition of cone beam computerized tomography, which is highly useful for imaging hard tissues of the head and neck in multiplanar slices, is ideal for visualizing decortications and periosteal changes.[41] Soft tissue changes can also be visualized in medical-grade CT scans by adding contrast medium (**Fig. 7**). The changes of early osteomyelitis are more clearly delineated and easier to interpret with CT images than with conventional radiography.[42] Its reconstruction capabilities can

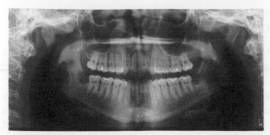

Fig. 6. Panoramic film of an acute osteomyelitis of number 17 site one month post extraction. Limited diagnostic changes are evident on this projection due to relatively long period required for lesion to affect bone density.

also be helpful in stereolythic model manufacturing and surgical treatment planning (**Figs. 8** and **9**).

MRI

Use of gadolinium as a contrast agent can show early osteomyelitis changes in tissue by highlighting nonspecific disturbances in tissue-blood interfaces, which are common in infection, inflammation, trauma, or tumors. The changes are most often noted in the soft tissuesand can also be noticed in the medullary portion of the affected bone.[43,44] In the T1-weighted images, these changes show low signal, whereas T2-weighted images show bright signal at the sites of inflammation because of increased water content. MRIs have a poor ability to analyze the condition and involvement of mandibular cortex particularly in early acute osteomyelitis.[6,43]

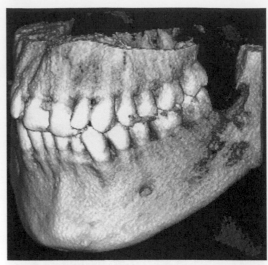

Fig. 8. 3D reconstruction of patient in **Fig. 6**, taken the same day but showing much greater osseous changes compared to the standard two dimensional modality.

Scintigraphy

The radioactive substances used to identify altered bone physiology are technetium 99m–labeled methylene diphosphonate, gallium 67, and indium 111. The most common scintigraphic agent is technetium 99m (**Fig. 10**), which is used to delineate increased bone turnover, and it is often coupled with the gallium 67 (**Fig. 11**) to distinguish the osteomyelitis lesions from tumor and trauma because gallium is sensitive to inflammatory

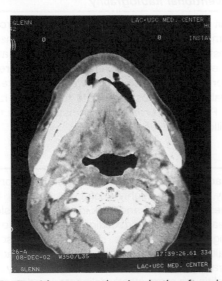

Fig. 7. CT with contrast showing both soft and hard tissue changes associated with chronic mandibular osteomyelitis.

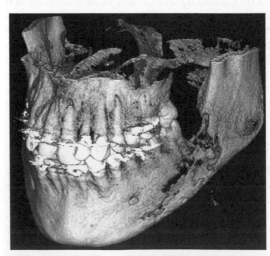

Fig. 9. Same patient as **Figs. 6** and **8** after additional two weeks of oral antibiotics therapy alone is showing the progression of the bone destruction and decalcification.

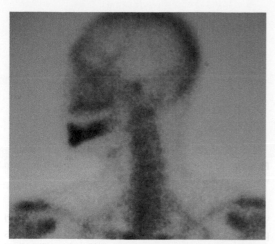

Fig. 10. Technetium scan showing uptake in the mandibular symphysis and body of an osteomyelitis patient.

changes.[6,40] The combined techniques have 98% sensitivity and can show changes as early as 3 days from the onset of infection.[1,40] Coupling of indium 111 is important when determining the activity of the lesion and the potential end point of therapy.[40,43] The downside of this technique is the exposure of the patient to a radiopharmaceutical. Therefore its use should be limited to cases in which a clear diagnostic benefit is expected.

PET/CT

The application of PET scan using fludeoxyglucose F 18 has shown promise in the identification of osteomyelitis in the jaws especially when applied with traditional CT. The 2 scanning modalities fuse together anatomic findings and a metabolic state finding in a real-time frame. Unlike other existing

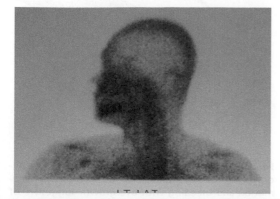

Fig. 11. Gallium scan showing similar mandibular involvement.

study modalities, a 3-dimensional image is obtained with high sensitivity and specificity.[45] Individual PET scans have a much higher rate of false-negative and false-positive results.[39] The linking of anatomic abnormalities with metabolic alterations is the key to pinpoint accuracy of the hybrid diagnostic modality in mandibular osteomyelitis.[46,47] The limited preliminary research data available show that the combined techniques have higher rates of specificity and sensitivity of traditional scintigraphy and leukocyte scintigraphy.[39,45] Because this is a relatively novel diagnostic approach, more research is needed to fully delineate all potential applications of this diagnostic and potentially surgically navigational technology. It is also hoped that as the PET scanning technology becomes more widely available and more economical, the access to this imaging will also improve for all practitioners in the community to routinely diagnose suspected osteomyelitis and measure real-time progress of the therapy.

INCIDENCE

Acute and chronic osteomyelitis are much more relevant in the mandible than in the maxilla. The literature has noted that the overall incidence of mandibular pyogenic osteomyelitis is up to 3 to 19 times greater than maxillary cases.[2,35,48–51] Historically, most cases in the maxilla were related to dental infections, orthognathic procedures, and malignancies.[1–3,52] The few documented infections were mostly associated with the dental support structures. However, with increase in bisphosphonate-related osteonecrosis cases, the maxillary skeleton involvement may become more prevalent.[52] In the mandible, the most common sites of osteomyelitis are the body, followed by the symphysis (**Figs. 12–14**), angle, ascending ramus, and condyle,[51] Both sexes are affected almost equally based on overall data from demographic studies.[6,32,35,50–52] Chronic osteomyelitis cases are more frequent after the second decade of life peaking, and this may correlate better with changes of the immune and vascular health of the adult and aging patient.[50,52] A rare infantile osteomyelitis variety can occur in newborn and infants and can involve the maxilla as well as the mandible. It is thought to have more of a hematogenous origin as a pathway for seeding of the bacterial infection in infants.[1,9]

CAUSE, PATHOGENESIS, AND MICROBIOLOGY

In most patients who develop osteomyelitis of the jaws, there is local spread of microflora into some wound connected to the medullary space. The

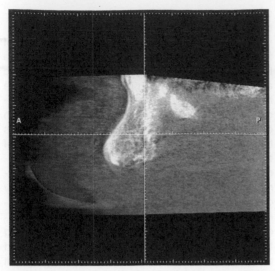

Fig. 12. Sagital cone beam CT showing mandibular symphysis osteomyelitis.

normal mixed microflora from oral and panfacial sinuses as well as skin in trauma cases has been implicated in the development of the disease. The bacteria associated with infected dentition, such as periodontal pathogens including *Staphylococcus aureus*, *Staphylococcus epidermidis*, Actinomyces, Prevotella species,[6,9,52] and Eikenella species, have been noted to be present in most chronic cases.[3,9,52] Candida infections were also noted in some of the cases of osteomyelitis.[52,53] The culturing of specific microorganism is very complex and often difficult to obtain in all clinical settings. Often, bone needs to be submitted in anaerobic medium or blood culture vials to prevent loss of anaerobic milieu. Gram staining and staining

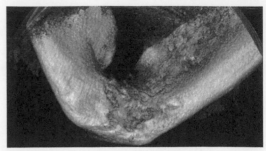

Fig. 14. 3D reconstruction of mandibular defect from worm's view.

with hematoxylin-eosin, van Gieson, Giemsa, and periodic acid–Schiff are the standard techniques helpful with early pathogen identification. The final results of culture and sensitivity test should guide the antimicrobial therapy after initial treatment with empirically derived regimens.[54–56]

Once seeded, the infections are thought to spread via the medullary marrow space and compromise the blood supply. This process is particularly damaging in the mandible, which has limited peripheral contributory supply and relies mainly on the inferior alveolar artery for blood flow. The affected bone is destroyed at a rapid rate in most suppurative cases with formation of sequestra and involucrum within cancellous and cortical portions.

Biopsied bone specimens from acute osteomyelitis have histologic findings of marrow spaces lined with neutrophilic granulocytes, necrotic bone, and inflammatory exudates (**Fig. 15**).[53] The increased pressure leads to further compromised vascularity and osteocyte necrosis. The sequestra become

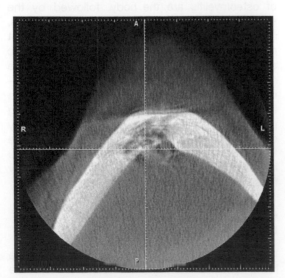

Fig. 13. Axial view of the same patient.

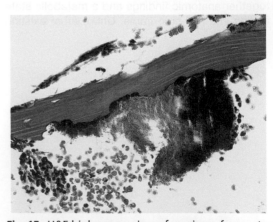

Fig. 15. H&E high power view of specimen from osteomyelitis showing sequestra of necrotic bone, inflammation and bleeding with overgrowth suggestive of actinomyces specie. (Courtesy of Paymon Parish Sedghizadeh, DDS, Los Angeles, CA.)

colonized with biofilm-forming microorganisms, which in turn leads to continued suppuration and chronicity of the process.

In chronic forms of osteomyelitis, the inflammatory infiltrate is composed of plasma cells, lymphocytes, and macrophages. Reactive bone formation is evident with irregular reversal lines seen similar to those of Paget disease.[53,55]

TREATMENT

Combined antimicrobial and surgical therapy is required in the management of all suppurative and chronic cases, with the exception of the infantile variety that may respond to intravenous medication alone.[1,3,32,54,56] The most important step in the process is a timely diagnosis before significant progression of the disease occurs. Early management reduces the morbidity and extent of surgical therapy required.

Other conditions including malignancies and metabolic disease should be excluded. The therapy is aimed at reducing bacterial challenge to the host's system. Surgical therapy physically reduces bacterial count but must be coupled with correction of any underlying medical conditions and well-targeted antimicrobial regimen. The addition of hyperbaric oxygen (HBO) therapy is also considered an important adjunct in swinging the pendulum in favor of host defensive and homeostatic systems.[57]

SURGICAL CORRECTION

The removal of necrotic bacteria–containing debris is accomplished through 3 distinct modalities. Sequestrectomy removes the localized free-standing areas of necrosis in the central area of infection (**Fig. 16**). Saucerization is more aggressive with the removal of adjacent bony cortices followed by exposure of the deeper layers of the medullary bone to allow for placement of packing materials and healing of soft tissues by secondary intention (**Fig. 17**). This approach can be useful in the early stages of disease and diseases of limited extent. It also allows for decompression of medullary cavity without significant removal of supporting structures of the mandible. The drawback is that this approach may be more likely to contaminate the specimen for culture and sensitivity testing because it is an all-transoral technique.[58]

Decortication is a more extensive approach, with intraoral and extraoral approaches possible, involving large broad bone removal of cortical bone, and it often requires lateralization of neurovascular bundle and rigid fixation to reduce pathologic fractures (**Fig. 18**). Primary closure is attempted over the site with mucoperiosteal covering of the newly exposed medullary space. This approach is advocated for larger lesions in advance acute or chronic osteomyelitis.[56]

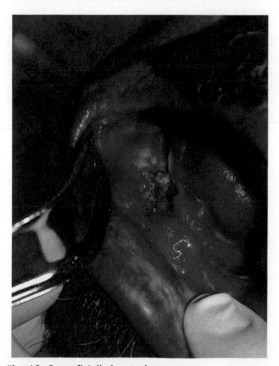

Fig. 16. Superficially located sequestra.

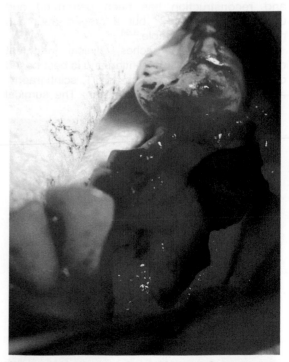

Fig. 17. Saucerization of mandibular defect maintains ridge continuity on lingual and buccal aspects of the body.

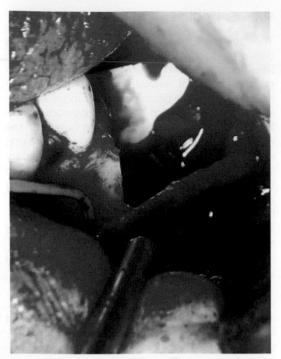

Fig. 18. Nerve laterization to allow for gross decortication of the defect.

In extensive defects or pathologic fractures, the site requires resection and subsequent reconstruction (**Fig. 19**). Early simultaneous resection and reconstruction has been performed and used by some,[54,59,60] but a staged approach may be more predictable.[3,56]

In all these approaches, clinical judgment directs the surgical intervention and is best based on imaging modalities such as CT, scintigraphy, and the new CT/PET fusion scan. The surgical end point of terminating resections at clinically viable bone stock with normal bone density and vascularity can be used when radiographic studies are not available or adequate (**Fig. 20**).

The wounds can be treated with acrylic beads laced with gentamicin as well as copious pulsed irrigation techniques using antimicrobial irrigants analogous to orthopedic long bone irrigation protocols.[48,56,61]

ANTIMICROBIAL THERAPY

As stated earlier, the initial antimicrobial therapy for osteomyelitis is based on using empirical coverage for the common causative pathogens. With treatment failures, a closer look at culture and sensitivity micropathology data when it becomes available is important. The first-line agents for this are clindamycin or amoxicillin/clavulanic acid combination regimens for minimum of 6 weeks.[62,63] Alternatively, for methicillin-susceptible S aureus infections, combination of flucloxacillin, ciprofloxacin, or levofloxacin with rifampin is advocated. For methicillin-resistant S aureus, combined vancomycin and rifampin therapy followed by oral ciprofloxacin or levofloxacin is considered appropriate. Peripherally inserted central catheter line should be placed and utilized during the IV therapy with frequent attention paid to condition and cleanliness of the access site (**Fig. 21**).

In cases of chronic osteomyelitis, similar regimens can be used, but intravenous medications can be limited to the initial 2 weeks of therapy and can then be followed by oral medication.[63] It is always a good idea to involve an infectious disease expert in coordinating the pharmacologic agent used in these more complex cases, especially in cases with past antibiotic therapeutic failures or when patient's multiple agent allergies are of concern.[3,54,56]

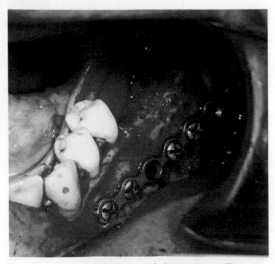

Fig. 19. Block resection and immediate iliac crest reconstruction of the body defect.

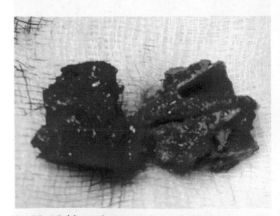

Fig. 20. Viable and necrotic bone from the osteomyelitic defect of the mandible showing differences in vascularity.

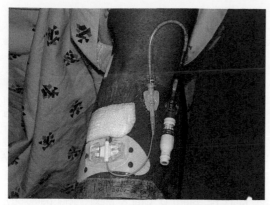

Fig. 21. Patient with a PICC line secured for IV antibiotic delivery.

HBO

An adjunct that has become available in the past 2 decades for therapy of osteomyelitis of the jaws is HBO therapy, which counters local hypoxia effects of medullary infections. For strictly anaerobic infections, the benefit of HBO is thought to be the greatest. However, no large-spectrum human prospective data studies support its use for early or acute osteomyelitis. Further, data must be gathered to demonstrate the value of this therapy in non–radiation-related osteomyelitis. In the meantime, it may be a modality to consider in refractory or host system incompetence cases.[3,54]

FOLLOW-UP AND CONTINUED CARE

The important concept in the management of infectious osteomyelitis is successful assessment of clinical interventions and the need for additional treatment in cases of failure or poor progress. The clinical picture is most important because it gives a real-time view of the process. Laboratory and radiographic values can be compared with baseline. At least a 2-year follow-up is important for acute osteomyelitis cases to ensure that no relapse is occurring. Reactivation of chronic osteomyelitis scan occurs even 10 years after primary therapy is concluded.[51] Reconstructive and regenerative procedures can be undertaken upon full resolution of the condition as long as the predisposing co–risk factors are well controlled. Otherwise, the patient may experience recurrence of the condition.

ACKNOWLEDGMENTS

Special thank you is extended to Ms Emily Williams who helped review this chapter along with my mother Dr Krystyna Zelichowski-Krakowiak who most notably also gave me this professional path and direction.

REFERENCES

1. Topazian RG. Osteomyelitis of the jaws. In: Topazian RG, Goldberg MH, editors. Oral and maxillofacial infections. Philadelphia: W.B.Saunders; 1994. p. 251–88.
2. Hudson JW. Osteomyelitis of the jaws: a 50-year perspective. J Oral Maxillofac Surg 1993;51(12):1294–301.
3. Marx RE. Chronic osteomyelitis of the jaws. Oral Maxillofac Surg Clin North Am 1991;3(2):376–81.
4. Panders AK, Hadders HN. Chronic sclerosing inflammations of the jaws. Osteomyelitis with fine-meshed trabecular structure and very dense sclerosing osteomyelitis. Oral Surg Oral Med Oral Pathol 1970;30(3):396–412.
5. Bernier S, Clermont S, Maranda G, et al. Osteomyelitis of the jaws. J Can Dent Assoc 1995;61(5):441–2.
6. Baltensperger M, Eyrich G. Osteomyelitis of the jaws: definitions and classification. In: Baltensperger M, Eyrich G, editors. Osteomyelitis of jaws. Berlin: Springer; 2009. p. 5–56.
7. Hunt TK, Halliday B, Knighton DR, et al. Impairment of antimicrobial functions in wounds: correction with oxygenation. In: Hunt TK, Hepppensatll RB, Pines E, et al, editors. Soft and hard tissue repair: biologic and clinical aspects. New York: Preger Scientific; 1984.
8. Mercuri LG. Acute osteomyelitis of the jaws. Oral Maxillofac Surg Clin North Am 1991;3(2):355–65.
9. Calhoun KH, Shapiro RD, Sternberg CM, et al. Osteomyelitis of the mandible. Arch Otolaryngol Head Neck Surg 1988;114:1157–62.
10. Zdinden R. Microbiology. In: Baltensperger M, Eyrich G, editors. Osteomyelitis of jaws. Berlin: Springer; 2009. p. 135–43.
11. Field EA, Speechley JA, Rotter E, et al. Dry socket incidence compared after a 12 year interval. Br J Oral Maxillofac Surg 1985;23(6):419–27.
12. Turner PS. A clinical study of 'dry socket'. Int J Oral Surg 1982;11(4):226–31.
13. Osborn TP, Frederickson G Jr, Small IA, et al. A prospective study of complications related to mandibular third molar surgery. J Oral Maxillofac Surg 1985;43(10):767–9.
14. Kolokythas A, Olech E, Miloro M. Alveolar osteitis: a comprehensive review of concepts and controversies. Int J Dent 2010;2010:1–10.
15. Nooroozi AR, Philbert RF. Modern concepts in understanding and management of the "dry socket" syndrome: comprehensive review of the literature. Oral Surg Oral Med Oral Pathol Oral Radiol Endod 2009;107(1):30–5.
16. Larsen PE. Alveolar osteitis after surgical removal of impacted mandibular third molars: identification of

the patient at risk. Oral Surg Oral Med Oral Pathol 1992;73(4):393–7.

17. Blum IR. Contemporary views on dry socket (alveolar osteitis): a clinical appraisal of standardization, aetiopathogenesis and management: a critical review. Int J Oral Maxillofac Surg 2002;31(3):309–17.

18. Swanson AE. Reducing the incidence of dry socket: a clinical appraisal. J Can Dent Assoc (Tor) 1966; 32(1):25–33.

19. Heasman PA, Jacobs DJ. A clinical investigation into the incidence of dry socket. Br J Oral Maxillofac Surg 1984;22(2):115–22.

20. Fridrich KL, Olson RA. Alveolar osteitis following surgical removal of mandibular third molars. Anesth Prog 1990;37(1):32–41.

21. Vezeau PJ. Dental extraction wound management: medicating post extraction sockets. J Oral Maxillofac Surg 2000;58(5):531–7.

22. Birn H. Etiology and pathogenesis of fibrinolytic alveolitis ('dry socket'). Int J Oral Surg 1973;2(5): 211–63.

23. Hindle MO, Gibbs A. The incidence of dry socket following the use of an occlusive dressing. J Dent 1977;5(4):288–93.

24. Nitzan DW. On the genesis of 'dry socket'. J Oral Maxillofac Surg 1983;41(11):706–10.

25. Rood JP, Murgatroyd J. Metronidazole in the prevention of 'dry socket'. Br J Oral Surg 1979;17(1):62–70.

26. Sweet JB, Butler DP. The relationship of smoking to localized osteitis. J Oral Surg 1979;37(10):732–5.

27. Catellani JE, Harvey S, Erickson SH, et al. Effect of oral contraceptive cycle on dry socket (localized alveolar osteitis). J Am Dent Assoc 1980;101(5): 777–80.

28. Schatz J-P, Fiore-Donno G, Henning G. Fibrinolytic alveolitis and its prevention. Int J Oral Maxillofac Surg 1987;16(2):175–83.

29. Summers L, Matz LR. Extraction wound sockets. Histological changes and paste packs–a trial. Br Dent J 1976;141(12):377–9.

30. Syrjanen SM, Syrjanen KJ. Influence of Alvogyl on the healing of extraction wound in man. Int J Oral Surg 1979;8(1):22–30.

31. Caso A, Hung L-K, Beirne OR. Prevention of alveolar osteitis with chlorhexidine: a meta-analytic review. Oral Surg Oral Med Oral Pathol Oral Radiol Endod 2005;99(2):155–9.

32. Wright DL, Kellman RM. Craniomaxillofacial bone infections: etiologies, distributions, and associated defects. In: Greenberg AM, Preim J, editors. Craniomaxillofacial reconstruction and corrective bone surgery principles of internal fixation using the AO/ASIF techniques. Berlin: Springer; 2002. p. 76–89.

33. Nelson LW, Lydiatt DD. Osteomyelitis of the head and neck. Nebr Med J 1987;72(5):154–63.

34. Bieluch VM, Gradner JG. Osteomyelitis of the skull, mandible and sternum. In: Jauregui LE, editor.

Diagnosis and management of bone infections. New York: Marcel Dekker; 1995. p. 109–33.

35. Koorbusch GF, Fotos P, Goll KT. Retrospective assessment of osteomyelitis: etiology, demographics, risk factors and management in 35 cases. Oral Surg Oral Med Oral Pathol 1992;74:149–54.

36. Roine I, Faingezicht I, Argueda A, et al. Serial serum C-reactive protein to monitor recovery from acute hematogenous osteomyelitis in children. Pediatr Infect Dis J 1994;93(1):59–62.

37. Goldstein BH. Unconventional dentistry Part IV Unconventional dental practices and products. J Can Dent Assoc 2000;66(10):564–8.

38. Marx RE, Stern D. Oral & Maxillofacial pathology: a rationale for diagnosis and treatment. Chicago: Quintessence Publishing Co. Inc; 2002. p. 885.

39. Terzic A, Goerres G. Diagnostic imaging-positron emission tomography, combined PET/CT. In: Baltensperger M, Eyrich G, editors. Osteomyelitis of jaws. Berlin: Springer; 2009. p. 113–9.

40. Hardt N, Hofer B, Baltensperger M. Diagnostic imaging scintigraphy. In: Baltensperger M, Eyrich G, editors. Osteomyelitis of jaws. Berlin: Springer; 2009. p. 95–112.

41. Prossor IM, Merkel KD, Fitzgerald RH, et al. Roentgenographic and radionuclide detection of musculoskeletal sepsis. In: Hughes SPF, Fitzgerald RH, editors. Musculoskeletal infections. Chicago: Year Book Medical Publishers Inc; 1986. p. 80–111.

42. Sculze D, Blessman B, Phlenz P, et al. Diagnostic criteria for detection of mandibular osteomyelitis using CBCT. Dentomaxillofac Radiol 2006;35(49): 232–5.

43. Schuknecht B. Diagnostic imaging- conventional radiology, computed tomography and magnetic resonance imaging. In: Baltensperger M, Eyrich G, editors. Osteomyelitis of jaws. Berlin: Springer; 2009. p. 57–94.

44. Weber PC, Seabold JE, Graham SM, et al. Evaluation of temporal and facial osteomyelitis by simultaneous in WBC/TC-99m-MDP bone SPECT scintigraphy and computer tomography scan. Otolaryngol Head Neck Surg 1995;113:36–41.

45. Tarmaat MF, Rajimakers PG, Scholten HJ, et al. J Bone Joint Surg Am 2005;87(1):2464–71.

46. Stumpe KD, Dazzi H, Schaffner A, et al. Infection imaging using whole body FDG-PET. Eur J Nucl Med 1998;25(9):1238–43.

47. Hakim SG, Brucker CW, Jacobsen Hernes D, et al. The value of FDG-PET and bone scintigraphy in primary diagnosis and follow up of patients with chronic osteomyelitis of the mandible. Int J Oral Maxillofac Surg 2006;35(9):809–16.

48. Chisholm BB, Lew D, Sadasivan IK. The use of tobramycin-impregnated polymetylmetacrylate beads in the treatment of osteomyelitis of the mandible. J Oral Maxillofac Surg 1993;51:444.

49. Kaneda T, Yamamoto H, Suzuki H, et al. A clinicoradiological study of maxillary osteomyelitis. J Nihon Univ Sch Dent 1989;31:464–9.

50. Adekeye EO, Cornah J. Osteomyelitis of the jaws: a review of 141 cases. Br J Oral Maxillofac Surg 1985;23:24–35.

51. Baltensperger MA. Retrospective analysis of 290 osteomyelitis cases treated in the past 30 years at the department of Craniomaxillofacial surgery Zurich with special recognition of the classification. Med Dissertion Zurich 2003;1:1–35.

52. Uche C, Mogyoros R, Chang A, et al. Osteomyelitis of the Jaw: a retrospective analysis. Int J Infect Dis 2009;7:2.

53. Bruder E, Jundt G, Eyrich G. Pathology of osteomyelitis. In: Baltensperger M, Eyrich G, editors. Osteomyelitis of jaws. Berlin: Springer; 2009. p. 121–33.

54. Kushner GM, Alpert B. Osteomyelitis and osteoradionecrosis. In: Miloro M, Gali GE, Larsen P, et al, editors. Peterson's principles of oral surgery. Hamilton (Canada): BC Decker; 2004. p. 317.

55. Eyrich GK, Langeenegger T, Bruder E, et al. Diffuse chronic sclerosis osteomyelitis and the sinovitis, acne, hyperostosis SAPHO syndrome in two sisters. Int J Oral Maxillofac Surg 2000;29:49–53.

56. Topazian RG. Osteomyelitis of jaws. In: Topazian RD, Goldberg MH, Hupp JR, editors. Oral & maxillofacial infections. 4th edition. Philadelphia: Saunders; 2002. p. 214–42.

57. Handschel J, Brussermann S, Deprrrich R, et al. Evaluation of hyperbaric oxygen in treatment of patients with osteomyelitis of the mandible. Mund-Kiefer Gesichtschir 2007;11(5):285–90.

58. Baltensperger M, Eyrich G. Osteomyelitis therapy-general consideration and surgical therapy. In: Baltensperger M, Eyrich G, editors. Osteomyelitis of jaws. Berlin: Springer; 2009. p. 145–78.

59. Obwegeser HL. Simultaneous resection of parts of the mandible via intraoral route in patients with and without gross infections. Oral Surg Oral Med Oral Pathol 1966;6:693–704.

60. Obwegeser HL, Sailer HF. Experiences with intraoral and partial resections of cases with mandibular osteomyelitis. J Maxillofac Surg 1978;6:34.

61. Alpert B, Colosi T, van Fraunhofer JA, et al. The in vivo behavior of gentamycin-PMMA beads in the maxillofacial region. J Oral Maxillofac Surg 1989;47:46.

62. Murry A. For how long should osteomyelitis be treated? In: Armstrong D, Cohen J, editors. Infectious disease. 2nd edition. London: Harcourt; 2005. p. 607–9.

63. Zimmirli W. Osteomyelitis therapy antibiotic therapy. Baltensperger M, Eyrich G, editors. Osteomyelitis of jaws. In: Baltensperger M, Eyrich G, editors. Osteomyelitis therapy-general consideration and surgical therapy. Berlin: Springer; 2009. p. 179–90.

Dentoalveolar Infections

Michael Lypka, MD, DMD[a,b,*],
Jeffrey Hammoudeh, MD, DDS[c]

KEYWORDS

- Dentoalveolar infection
- Maxillofacial infection
- Odontogenic infection

Dentoalveolar infections represent a spectrum of conditions ranging from localized periodontal abscesses, to deep neck space infections, to the most severe case of necrotizing fasciitis. The oral and maxillofacial surgeon is faced with managing all these conditions, from the most mundane to the life threatening. A topic addressed by several investigators over the years, and perhaps an uninspiring one to some with little new information, it has never been more important to be adept in diagnosing and managing dentoalveolar infections. A recent report by Sepannen and colleagues[1] has shown a disturbing trend toward an increased severity of maxillofacial infections in the last 10 years in 1 hospital district, with a trend toward more medically complicated patients. The subject of dentoalveolar infections allows oral and maxillofacial surgeons to integrate their knowledge of anatomy, medicine, microbiology, anesthesiology, pharmacology, and surgery into a diagnostic and therapeutic plan that can be not only intellectually stimulating but also potentially life saving.

PATIENT ASSESSMENT

As in all patient encounters, evaluation of a patient with a dentoalveolar infection should begin with a good history and physical examination, and a clinical impression of the severity of the infection should be apparent immediately, without the need for additional laboratory or radiologic data. The history should include the onset, duration, and type of symptoms, as well as previous therapies. It is important to ascertain if the patient is having any odynophagia, dysphagia, or respiratory difficulties. The patient's medical history, including a history of diabetes, renal disorders, and immunodeficiencies, can assist the clinician in assessing the host's ability to fight the infection. In some cases, the oral and maxillofacial surgeon may be the first to diagnose diabetes because the stress of a dentoalveolar infection unmasks glucose intolerance. Current medications, including chemotherapy and steroid therapy, and a history of alcohol and drug abuse are also important historical information.

The physical examination begins with an assessment of the vital signs, followed by a thorough examination of the patient. Tachycardia suggests dehydration or pain, or it may be the result of increased temperature. Hypotension would be the most concerning, suggesting a dehydrated, septic patient. The patient with a severe dentoalveolar infection has a typical toxic appearance. The head posture of the patient should be assessed, with the sniffing position and accessory respiratory muscle use suggesting upper airway obstruction from airway swelling. The quality of the patient's

The authors have nothing to disclose.

a Division of Pediatric Plastic and Craniofacial Surgery, Department of Pediatric Surgery, University of Texas Medical School at Houston, 6431 Fannin Street, MSB 5.281, Houston, TX 77030, USA

b Division of Plastic and Reconstructive Surgery, Department of Surgery, University of Texas Medical School at Houston, 6431 Fannin Street, MSB 5.281, Houston, TX 77030, USA

c Division of Plastic and Maxillofacial Surgery, Department of Surgery, Children's Hospital Los Angeles, Keck School of Medicine, University of Southern California, 4650 Sunset Boulevard MS 96, Los Angeles, CA 90027, USA

* Corresponding author. Division of Pediatric Plastic and Craniofacial Surgery, Department of Pediatric Surgery, University of Texas Medical School at Houston, 6431 Fannin Street, MSB 5.281, Houston, TX 77030.
E-mail address: michael.a.lypka@uth.tmc.edu

Oral Maxillofacial Surg Clin N Am 23 (2011) 415–424
doi:10.1016/j.coms.2011.04.010
1042-3699/11/$ – see front matter © 2011 Elsevier Inc. All rights reserved.

voice, as in a "hot potato" voice, would indicate glottal swelling. The patient's maximal incisal opening is an important physical finding, with a limited opening less than 30 mm indicating involvement of the masticatory muscles, as in a masticator, or lateral pharyngeal space infection. Limited mouth opening should alert the practitioner to a more severe infection with a greater probability of having a difficult intubation, if necessary.[2] Floor of mouth elevation and uvular deviation indicating sublingual and lateral pharyngeal space infection, respectively, should be noted on intraoral examination. The condition of the dentition should be assessed, and the source of the infection sought. Swelling in the vicinity of the body of the mandible should be carefully assessed. A palpable inferior border suggests a buccal space infection, amenable to intraoral drainage, whereas swelling extending inferior to it would suggest submandibular space infection, requiring extraoral drainage.

Radiographic imaging is a useful aid in diagnosing and guiding surgical therapy for dentoalveolar infections. The gold standard for imaging of maxillofacial infections, especially deep anatomic space infections, is computed tomography (CT) with intravenous contrast.[3] The contrast enhances the ability to visualize abscess cavities, assess lymphadenopathy, and visualize vascular structures, such as jugular venous thrombosis. Although magnetic resonance imaging is useful for localization of soft tissue abscess,[4] the length of the study makes it a less-desirable option, especially in a patient with possible impending airway compromise. Ultrasonography may be used to differentiate cellulitis from abscess in superficial neck infections, but its role in deep neck space infections is limited.[5,6] Lateral plain films to assess retropharyngeal involvement are largely of historical interest, given the availability and speed of the current CT scanners. Certainly, an orthopantomogram is a useful radiograph to assess the dentition and determine the source of the infection.

Laboratory workup should consist of a complete blood cell count with differential and basic metabolic panels. C-reactive protein may be used as a marker to assess the severity of infection[7] and response to treatment. Typically, blood cultures yield negative results in patients with dentoalveolar infections and are not indicated. Culture and sensitivity testing should be a routine practice during surgical drainage to guide antibiotic therapy, especially given nonresponse rates of 21% with empirical penicillin therapy in the inpatient setting in 1 report.[8] Cultures should preferably be aspirates and transported to the laboratory within 2 hours.

With completion of a history and physical examination, and perhaps before completion of a thorough assessment, airway management must be the primary consideration in managing a patient with dentoalveolar infection. Depending on the severity of airway compromise, close clinical observation, intubation, or tracheotomy are all considerations for airway management. When intubation is deemed necessary for airway protection, awake fiberoptic techniques are preferable. In other cases, tracheotomy may be the best alternative. Tracheotomy may result in earlier transfer out of the intensive care unit and a reduced hospital stay when compared with intubation in patients with deep neck space infections.[9]

NATURAL HISTORY OF PROGRESSION

Dentoalveolar infections arise from either periapical or periodontal sources. In the case of periapical infection, pulpal necrosis resulting from dental caries allows invasion of bacteria into the periapical tissue. In the case of periodontal infection, deep periodontal pockets allow inoculation of bacteria into the underlying soft tissues. Periapical infection is by far the most common cause of odontogenic infections. Once bacteria gain access to the periapical bone, 2 possibilities may arise. Either a chronic process ensues, such as periapical cyst or granuloma formation, osteomyelitis, or fistula formation, or an acute phenomenon takes place. An acute process may take the form of cellulitis, dentoalveolar abscess, fascial space infection, or, in the worst case, necrotizing fasciitis. Bacteria from the periodontal or periapical soft tissues may rarely spread hematogenously, as evidenced by infection at distant anatomic sites such as the spine,[10] liver, or brain.[11]

LOCAL ANATOMIC CONSIDERATIONS

Periapical infections that perforate the cortical bone, usually at the thinnest site, localize based on the relationship of the roots of the teeth to the origins and insertions of facial muscles to the maxillary and mandibular alveoli (Fig. 1). An understanding of these relationships is essential in diagnosing and predicting the spread of dentoalveolar infections. The buccinator muscle inserts onto the most superior and inferior portions of the alveolar processes of the maxilla and mandible, respectively. Bony destruction with spread of infection above the superior attachment or below the inferior attachment results in a buccal space infection. Infectious escape within these insertions results in a vestibular space infection. The mylohyoid muscle arises from the mylohyoid line of the mandible, and its relationship to the root apices of the lower molar and premolar teeth defines

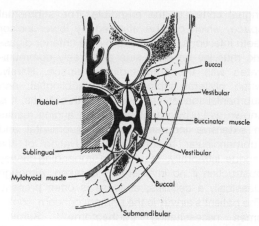

Fig. 1. Direction of spread of infection from maxillary and mandibular teeth. (*From* Goldberg MH, Topazian RG. Odontogenic infections and deep fascial space infections of dental origin. In: Topazian RG, Goldberg MH, editors. Oral and maxillofacial infections. 2nd edition. Philadelphia: WB Saunders; 1987. p. 170; with permission.)

spread of infection to the submandibular or sublingual spaces. The mylohyoid line slopes superiorly as it travels posteriorly. Therefore, lower second and third molar teeth infections tend to spread into the submandibular space because their root apices are below the muscle origin, whereas premolar infections tend to spread into the sublingual space, their root apices being cephalad to the mylohyoid line. Maxillary sinusitis is also a possible sequela of apical infections of the maxillary molars because of their intimate relationship to the floor of the maxillary sinus.

FASCIAL ANATOMY OF SPACE INFECTIONS

An understanding of head and neck fascial relationships is paramount in truly understanding the presentation, spread, and surgical treatment of dentoalveolar infections. The study of fascial layers of the head and neck can be a confusing topic because of the complex anatomy in the region and the use of different nomenclatures to describe the same anatomy. The authors try to make some sense of the fascial layers in this article. The fascia of the head and neck, in simple terms, is classified into superficial and deep. The superficial fascia of the head and neck is the layer of fascia closest to the skin and has different names depending on the anatomic area. In the temporal area, it is known as the temporoparietal fascia or superficial temporal fascia. As one progresses caudad, the temporoparietal fascia becomes continuous with the superficial musculoaponeurotic system (SMAS), the fascial system that envelops the muscles of facial expression. The SMAS then becomes continuous with the fascia enveloping the platysma muscle in the neck. The significance of the superficial fascia in head and neck infections is relevant mainly to superficial skin infections and, rarely, dentoavleolar infections that may make their way through this fascia to the skin surface. The superficial borders of the buccal, submandibular, and submental spaces are defined by the superficial fascia.

The deep fascia of the neck is further subdivided into superficial, middle, and deep layers. The superficial layer of the deep cervical fascia sometimes called the investing fascia, not to be confused with the superficial fascia described earlier, completely encircles the neck and invests the trapezius and sternocleidomastoid muscles, as well as the submandibular glands. Traveling cephalad, the superficial layer of the deep cervical fascia splits to envelop the masseter, lateral to the mandible, and the medial pterygoid, medial to the mandible. The parotidomasseteric fascia is another name for the superficial layer of the deep cervical fascia enveloping the parotid gland, whereas the temporalis fascia represents a continuation of this fascia in the temporal region. The superficial layer of the deep cervical fascia in the head, therefore, defines the masticator space, made up of submasseteric, pterygomandibular, and superficial and deep temporal spaces.

The middle layer of deep cervical fascia consists of a muscular division, which surrounds the strap muscles of the neck, and a visceral division, surrounding the thyroid, trachea, and esophagus. The visceral division is more commonly named the pretracheal fascia anteriorly and the buccopharyngeal fascia posteriorly, which lines the deep surface of the pharyngeal constrictors. The middle layer of the deep cervical fascia is continuous with the pericardium and thoracic trachea and esophagus in the chest.

The deep layer of the deep cervical fascia consists of the prevertebral and alar fascia. The prevertebral fascia invests the posterior neck muscles and vertebral bodies and extends from the base of the skull to the coccyx. The alar fascia is a thin wispy layer of fascia that lies between the prevertebral fascia posteriorly and the buccopharyngeal fascia anteriorly. It extends inferiorly from the base of the skull and, unlike the prevertebral fascia, ends at T2 level, where it fuses with the buccopharyngeal fascia of the middle layer of the deep cervical fascia. The carotid sheath is made up of all 3 portions of the deep cervical fascia, including superficial, middle, and deep layers, a reason for potential thrombosis of the jugular vein in adjacent fascial space infections. A good example of this phenomenon is Lemierre syndrome,[12] in which oropharyngeal infection spreads to the internal jugular vein, thrombosing it.

Between the deep layers of fascia exist potential spaces for routes of spread of infection (**Fig. 2**). The retropharyngeal space lies between the buccopharyngeal fascia and alar fascia, whereas danger space No. 4,[13] often incorrectly named the prevertebral space, takes up the space between the alar and prevertebral fascia. A potential space between the vertebral bodies and the prevertebral fascia makes up the prevertebral space. The significance of the anatomy here illustrates how a dentoalveolar infection of the lateral pharyngeal space can travel to the thorax by spreading to the retropharyngeal space tracking caudad, and piercing the weak alar fascia into danger space No. 4, gaining access to the mediastinum.

SPECIFIC HEAD AND NECK SPACE INFECTIONS

The authors briefly describe common head and neck space infections, keeping in mind the fascial relationships discussed earlier. In the maxilla, the canine space is involved, usually from a canine tooth, when infection erodes through the alveolar bone superior to the origin of the levator anguli oris muscle (**Fig. 3**). Swelling of the midface on the affected side occurs, often with extension superiorly, resulting in a preseptal cellulitis. The buccal space is superficial to the buccinator muscle and is lined externally by the skin and superficial fascia of the face (**Fig. 4**). This space may be affected by maxillary or, less commonly, mandibular teeth when infection erodes outside the insertion of the muscle. The infratemporal space lies posterior to the maxilla and can be involved when a maxillary third molar becomes infected. It is significant in that hematogenous spread of infection through the adjacent valveless pterygoid plexus to the cavernous sinus can result in cavernous sinus thrombosis,[14] a life-threatening infection. A similar pathway of spread to the orbit can result in orbital infection.[15,16]

The spaces of the mandible adjacent the teeth include the submandibular, submental, and sublingual spaces (**Fig. 5**). The sublingual space lies between the floor of the mouth and mylohyoid muscle, and is typically affected by infections of premolar teeth or spread from the adjacent submandibular space. The submandibular space lies between the mylohyoid muscle and the overlying skin and superficial fascia. Its medial border is formed by the anterior and posterior digastric muscles (**Fig. 6**). It is involved when the lower second and third molar abscesses perforate the

lingual cortex of the mandible. The submental space, which can be affected by lower incisor teeth infections, is bounded by the anterior digastric muscles on each side and freely communicates with the submandibular space. Rarely, when bilateral submandibular, sublingual, and submental spaces are involved with cellulitis, it is known as Ludwig angina. Ludwig angina results in extensive induration of the submental and submandibular regions, with elevation of the tongue intraorally, resulting in impending airway obstruction if no intervention is taken. Although classically a cellulitis, abscess is often present. The patient's airway is the primary concern, sometimes necessitating tracheotomy.[17] Surgical drainage is the preferred treatment.

The masticator space is defined by the superficial layer of the deep cervical fascia because it envelops the mandible and masticatory muscles. It is made up of the submasseteric space, bounded by the masseter muscle laterally, the pterygomandibular space, bounded by the medial pterygoid muscle medially, and the deep and superficial temporal spaces, surrounding the temporalis muscle superiorly extending up from the coronoid process of the mandible. Spread of infection to the deep temporal space from an abscessed molar can therefore explain temporal bone osteomyelitis, as reported by Adams and Bryant.[18] The lateral pharyngeal space is an inverted cone extending from the base of the skull to the hyoid bone inferiorly. It is bounded laterally by the medial pterygoid muscle and medially by the superior pharyngeal constrictor or buccopharyngeal fascia. It is split into anterior and posterior compartments by styloid musculature, the posterior of which contains the carotid sheath and cranial nerves IX through XII. Spread of infection posteriorly into any of these spaces causes significant trismus, and in the case of extension into the posterior compartment of the lateral pharyngeal space, cranial nerve involvement, Horner syndrome, or jugular venous thrombosis. Spread of infection to the lateral pharyngeal space, as discussed in the Fascial Anatomy of Space Infections section, can allow extension into the retropharyngeal space, subsequently gaining entry to the mediastinum.

OTHER DENTOALVEOLAR INFECTIONS

In the most severe form, dentoalveolar infections can progress to necrotizing fasciitis, an aggressive, typically polymicrobial, infection resulting in liquefaction of underlying fat and fascia. With a mortality of up to 60%,[19] early recognition and aggressive operative intervention are necessary.[20]

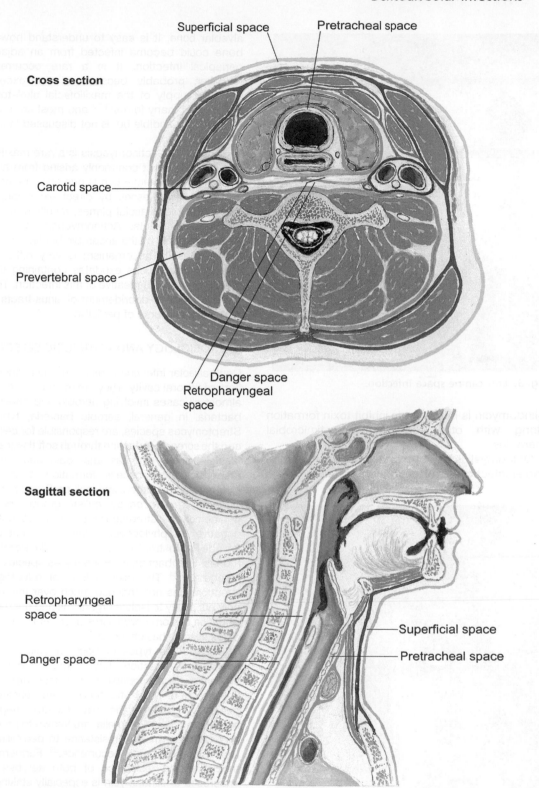

Fig. 2. Fascial spaces of the neck (*red line*) investing fascia (superficial layer of the deep cervical fascia), (*blue line*) pretracheal fascia (visceral division of the middle layer of the deep cervical fascia), (*green line*) buccopharyngeal fascia (visceral division of the middle layer of the deep cervical fascia), (*orange line*) alar fascia (deep layer of the deep cervical fascia), (*brown line*) carotid sheath, (*yellow line*) prevertebral fascia (deep layer of the deep cervical fascia), (*purple line*) muscular division of the middle layer of the deep cervical fascia. (*From* Netter illustration Elsevier Inc. All rights reserved. Available at www.netterimages.com; with permission.)

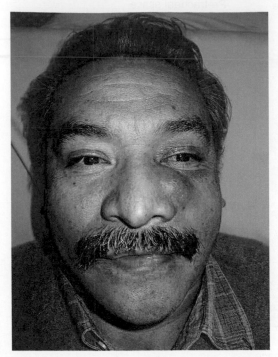

Fig. 3. Left canine space infection.

Clindamycin is indicated to inhibit toxin formation along with other combination antimicrobial therapies.

Osteomyelitis is another rare sequela of dentoalveolar infections. The teeth being embedded in the

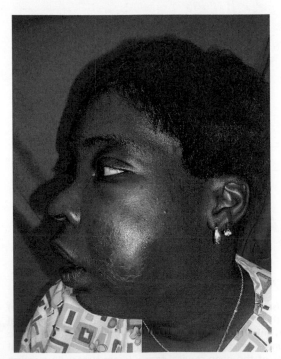

Fig. 4. Left buccal space infection.

alveolar bone, it is easy to understand how the bone could become infected from an adjacent periapical infection. It is a rare occurrence, however, probably because of the excellent vascular supply of the maxillofacial skeleton. It can exist in many forms[21,22] and most commonly affects the mandible but is not discussed in detail in this article.

Cervicofacial actinomycosis is a rare maxillofacial infection most commonly arising from an infected tooth. The infection is primarily one of soft tissue and progresses by direct extension, not following typical fascial planes, resulting in cutaneous sinus tracts. Actinomycosis is caused most commonly by the anaerobic bacteria *Actinomyces israelii*. The organism is very difficult to culture but produces exudates containing sulfur granules, highly suggestive of this infection. Treatment consists of debridement of sinus tracts and a prolonged course of penicillin.

MICROBIOLOGY AND ANTIBIOTIC SELECTION

Dentoalveolar infections arise from the indigenous flora of the oral cavity. They are mixed infections in almost all cases involving aerobic and anaerobic bacteria. In general, aerobic bacteria, typically Streptomyces species, are responsible for cellulitis and the spread of infection through soft tissues and fascial planes, whereas anaerobic bacteria are responsible for abscess formation. Commonly isolated aerobic organisms include *Streptococcus viridans*, *Streptococcus milleri* group species, β- hemolytic streptococcus, and coagulase-negative staphylococci. Common anaerobes include Peptostreptococcus, Prevotella, Porphyromonas, Fusobacterium, Bacteroides species, and Eikenella.[23,24] The microbiology of odontogenic infections has not changed much over the years, only our ability to isolate organisms and our reclassification of some organisms such as the Bacteroides species has changed.[25]

Whereas the types of bacteria cultured from odontogenic infections have remained constant, the antibiotic susceptibility of various organisms has changed. Most streptococci are sensitive to penicillin.[26] However, the anaerobic gram-negative bacteria, such as Prevotella, are known to produce β-lactamases, making resistance to penicillins an increasingly common occurrence.[27] Furthermore, the increasing resistance of both aerobes and anaerobes to clindamycin is especially striking, as highlighted in the recent article by Poeschl and colleagues[28] Recommendations for empirical therapy, based on available data, are difficult to make. Penicillin remains the antibiotic of choice for outpatient management of less-severe infections,

Sagittal section through neck

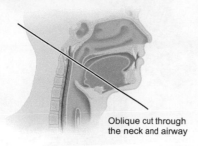

Oblique cut through
the neck and airway

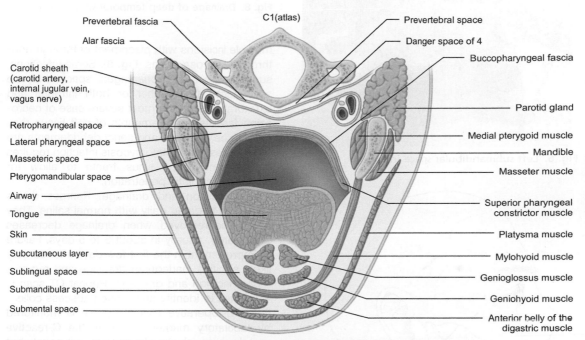

Prevertebral fascia

Alar fascia

Carotid sheath
(carotid artery,
internal jugular vein,
vagus nerve)

Retropharyngeal space

Lateral pharyngeal space

Masseteric space

Pterygomandibular space

Airway

Tongue

Skin

Subcutaneous layer

Sublingual space

Submandibular space

Submental space

C1(atlas)

Prevertebral space

Danger space of 4

Buccopharyngeal fascia

Parotid gland

Medial pterygoid muscle

Mandible

Masseter muscle

Superior pharyngeal
constrictor muscle

Platysma muscle

Mylohyoid muscle

Genioglossus muscle

Geniohyoid muscle

Anterior belly of the
digastric muscle

Fig. 5. Anatomy of maxillofacial space infections. (*From* Girn J, Jo C. Ludwig's angina. In: Bagheri S, Jo C, editors. Clinical review of oral and maxillofacial surgery. St Louis: Mosby; 2008. p. 71; with permission.)

whereas clindamycin is a reasonable choice in the penicillin allergic patient. For more severe infections managed in the hospital, ampicillin/clavulanic acid, with excellent activity against anaerobic bacterial β-lactamases, or moxifloxacin,[29] a fluorquinolone with efficacious broad-spectrum coverage, are good options. Regardless of the empirical choice, surgical therapy is the primary treatment modality for dentoalveolar infections and antibiotic therapy must be guided by the culture and sensitivity testing.

SURGICAL THERAPY

The primary goal of surgical therapy for dentoalveolar infections is to drain the infection and remove the source of infection, usually by extracting the offending tooth at the same time

as the incision and drainage. Abscess, without question, requires incision and drainage, whereas the surgical management of cellulitis is more controversial. It is the opinion of these authors, and others,[30] that there is benefit to aggressive surgical management of all fascial spaces affected by cellulitis because it alters the bacterial milieu and hastens the resolution of infection.

A few guiding principles of surgical drainage include placing the incision in healthy mucosa or skin and in an aesthetic area, if possible; obtaining gravity-dependent drainage; and performing blunt dissection during drainage to avoid damage to adjacent vital structures.[31] The specific sites of drainage for each particular space infection are not discussed in detail in this article but are shown in **Figs. 7** and **8**. Many infections may require

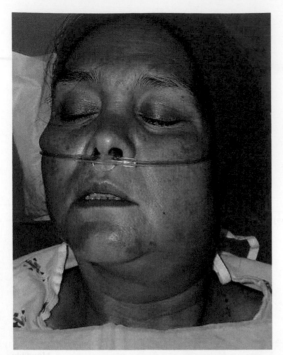

Fig. 6. Left submandibular space infection.

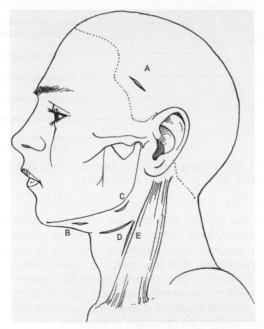

Fig. 7. Incision placement for extraoral drainage of deep neck space infections. (A) Superficial or deep temporal; (B) submental or submandibular; (C) submandibular, submasseteric, or pterygomandibular; (D) lateral pharyngeal space and upper portion of retropharyngeal space; (E) retropharyngeal space and carotid sheath (may be combined with D) incisions. (From Flynn TR. Surgical management of orofacial infections. Atlas Oral Maxillofac Surg Clin North Am 2000;8(1):85; with permission.)

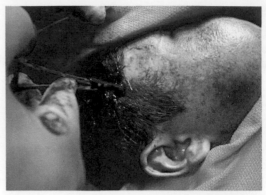

Fig. 8. Drainage of deep temporal space infection.

multiple incisions with placement of through-and-through Penrose drains (Fig. 9). Some infections, such as the lateral pharyngeal space, may be approached from either or both intraoral and extraoral sites. In the most severe case of necrotizing fasciitis, large amounts of soft tissue may have to be debrided and serial debridements are often necessary. Actinomycosis infection requires debridement of all sinus tracts to allow for adequate antibiotic penetration.

After incision and drainage, Penrose drains should be irrigated daily with normal saline. They should be removed when drainage decreases significantly, usually in about 3 to 5 days. Failure of improvement in the first few days after surgery likely signifies inadequate drainage and requires repeat incision and drainage. Repeat CT scan is warranted to identify any missed abscess collection. Postoperative clinical course is monitored by laboratory markers such as the C-reactive protein or serial complete blood cell count, but none of these markers can replace good clinical judgment.

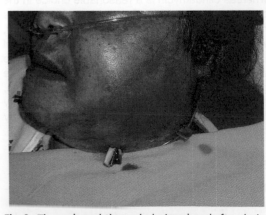

Fig. 9. Through-and-through drains placed after drainage of a submandibular space infection.

SUMMARY

Dentoalveolar infections represent a wide spectrum of conditions, from simple localized abscesses to deep neck space infections. The initial assessment of the patient with a dentoalveolar infection requires considerable clinical skill and experience, and determines the need for further airway management or emergent surgical therapy. Knowledge of head and neck fascial space anatomy is essential in diagnosing, understanding spread, and surgically managing these infections. Whereas the microbiology of dentoalveolar infection has remained constant, antibiotic resistance profiles continue to change. Surgical drainage is the hallmark of treating all dentoalveolar infections. Oral and maxillofacial surgeons must make use of their wide spectrum of clinical skill and knowledge to effectively evaluate and treat patients with dentoalveolar infections.

REFERENCES

1. Seppanen L, Rautemaa R, Lindqvist C, et al. Changing clinical features of odontogenic maxillofacial infections. Clin Oral Investig 2010;14:459–65.
2. Frerk CM. Predicting difficult intubation. Anaesthesia 1993;46:1005.
3. Lazor JB, Cunningham MJ, Eavey RD, et al. Comparison of computed tomography and surgical findings in deep neck space infections. Otolaryngol Head Neck Surg 1994;111:746.
4. Schuknecht B, Stergiou G, Graetz K. Masticator space abscess derived from odontogenic infection, imaging manifestation, and pathways of extension depicted by CT and MR in 30 patients. Eur Radiol 2008;18:1972–9.
5. Peleg M, Heyman Z, Ardekian L, et al. The use of ultrasonography as a diagnostic tool for superficial fascial space infections. J Oral Maxillofac Surg 1998;56:1129–31.
6. Bassiony M, Yang J, Abel-Monem TM, et al. Exploration of ultrasonography in assessment of fascial space spread of odontogenic infection. Oral Surg Oral Med Oral Pathol Oral Radiol Endod 2009;107: 861–9.
7. Ylijoki S, Suuronen R, Jousimies-Somer H, et al. Differences in patients with and without the need for intensive care due to severe odontogenic infections. J Oral Maxillofac Surg 2001;59:867–72.
8. Flynn TR, Shanti RM, Levi MH, et al. Severe odontogenic infections, part 1: prospective report. J Oral Maxillofac Surg 2006;64:1093.
9. Potter JK, Herford AS, Ellis E. Tracheotomy versus endotracheal intubation for airway management in deep neck space infections. J Oral Maxillofac Surg 2001;60:349–54.
10. Dhariwal DK, Patton DW, Gregory MC. Epidural spinal abscess following dental extraction–a rare and potentially fatal complication. Br J Oral Maxillofac Surg 2003;41:56–8.
11. Wagner KW, Schon R, Schumacher M, et al. Case report: brain and liver abscesses caused by oral infection with Streptococcus intermedius. Oral Surg Oral Med Oral Pathol Oral Radiol Endod 2006;102: e21–3.
12. Malis DD, Busaidy KF, Marchena JM. Lemierre Syndrome and descending necrotizing mediastinitis following dental extraction. J Oral Maxillofac Surg 2008;66:1720–5.
13. Grodinsky M, Holoyoke EA. The fasciae and fascial spaces of head, neck, and adjacent regions. Am J Anat 1938;63:367.
14. Colbert S, Cameron M, Williams J. Septic thrombosis of the cavernous sinus and dental infection. Br J Oral Maxillofac Surg 2010 Aug 4. [Epub ahead of print].
15. Munoz-Guerra MF, Gonzalez-Garcia R, Capote AL, et al. Subperiosteal abscess of the orbit; an unusual complication of third molar surgery. Oral Surg Oral Med Oral Pathol Oral Radiol Endod 2006;102:e9–13.
16. Kim IK, Kim JR, Jang KS, et al. Orbital abscess from an odontogenic infection. Oral Surg Oral Med Oral Pathol Oral Radiol Endod 2007;103:e1–6.
17. Pahiscar A, Har-El G. Deep neck abscesses: a retrospective review of 210 cases. Ann Otol Rhinol Laryngol 2001;110:1051.
18. Adams JR, Bryant DG. Cranial osteomyelitis: a late complication of a dental infection. Br J Oral Maxillofac Surg 2008;46:673–4.
19. Roberson JB, Harper JL, Jauch EC. Mortality associated with cervicofacial necrotizing fasciitis. Oral Surg Oral Med Oral Pathol Oral Radiol Endod 1996;82:264–7.
20. Caccamese JF, Coletti DP. Deep neck space infections: clinical considerations in aggressive disease. Oral Maxillofac Surg Clin North Am 2008;20:367–80.
21. Coviello V, Stevens MR. Contemporary concepts in the treatment of chronic osteomyelitis. Oral Maxillofac Surg Clin North Am 2007;19:523–34.
22. Montonen M, Lindqvist C. Diagnosis and treatment of diffuse sclerosing osteomyelitis of the jaws. Oral Maxillofac Surg Clin North Am 2003;15:69–78.
23. Rega AJ, Aziz SR, Ziccardi VB. Microbiology and antibiotic sensitivities of head and neck space infections of odontogenic origin. J Oral Maxillofac Surg 2006;64:1377–80.
24. Brook I. Microbiology and management of peritonsillar, retropharyngeal, and parapharyngeal abscesses. J Oral Maxillofac Surg 2004;62:1545–50.
25. Haug R. The changing microbiology of maxillofacial infections. Oral Maxillofac Surg Clin North Am 2003; 15:1–15.

26. Kuriyama T, Karasawa T, Nakagawa K, et al. Bacteriologic features and antimicrobial susceptibility in isolates from orofacial odontogenic infections. Oral Surg Oral Med Oral Pathol Oral Radiol Endod 2000;90:600–8.

27. Lewis MA, Parkhurst CL, Douglas CW, et al. Prevalence of penicillin resistant bacteria in acute suppurative oral infection. J Antimicrob Chemother 1995;35:785–91.

28. Poeschl PW, Spusta L, Russmeuller G, et al. Antibiotic susceptibility and resistance of the odontogenic microbiological spectrum and its clinical impact on severe deep space head and neck infections. Oral Surg Oral Med Oral Pathol Oral Radiol Endod 2010;11:151–6.

29. Warnke PH, Becker ST, Springer IN, et al. Penicillin compared with other advanced broad spectrum antibiotics regarding antibacterial activity against oral pathogens isolated from odontogenic abscesses. J Craniomaxillofac Surg 2008;36:462–7.

30. Flynn TR. Surgical management of orofacial infections. Atlas Oral Maxillofac Surg Clin North Am 2000;8:77–100.

31. Topazian RG, Goldberg MH. Odontogenic infections and deep fascial space infections of dental origin. In: Topazian RG, editor. Oral and maxillofacial infections. 4th edition. Philadelphia: WB Saunders Company; 2002.

Craniocervical Necrotizing Fasciitis Resulting from Dentoalveolar Infection

Joseph Brunworth, MD[a], Terry Y. Shibuya, MD[a,b],*

KEYWORDS

- Dentoalveolar complications
- Craniocervical necrotizing fasciitis • Neck infection

Dental infections frequently occur and are routinely managed by local dental therapies and antibiotics. Unfortunately, infections can spread beyond the dentoalveolar ridge and extend into the soft tissues of the neck and face. In instances where there is extension of infection into the soft tissue and fascial compartment of the neck and face, this necessitates hospital admission, surgical debridement, intravenous antibiotics, and dental extractions.

In the most severe form of dental infection, necrotizing fasciitis can develop, which is commonly recognized by the public as an infection of "flesh-eating bacteria." Certain individuals are more susceptible to developing such severe infections, including patients who have delayed dental infection treatment; those who have comorbid health conditions, such as diabetes mellitus, alcoholism, and malnutrition; and those who are immunocompromised because of either infection (AIDS) or cancer.[1] This is the most severe form of a dental infection and, if not recognized immediately and treated quickly, it can result in significant morbidities and ultimately death.

Necrotizing fasciitis of the head and neck is a rare but potentially lethal disease process involving infection and subsequent destruction of fascial planes beneath the dermal skin layer. Left untreated, this disease leads to thoracic extension, sepsis, and death within a short period of time. Only a small percentage of necrotizing fasciitis involves the head or neck; this is termed "craniocervical necrotizing fasciitis" (CCNF). Often polymicrobial in nature, this aggressive infection causes local ischemia because of vascular occlusion, and local anesthesia because of neural damage. Of significant interest, both the literature and the authors' experience show that most CCNF arises from dental infections (**Table 1**).[1-11] This is important to understand, considering the high frequency of dental infections in the general population. Although rare, necrotizing fasciitis of the head and neck is a deadly condition that dentists, oral maxillofacial surgeons, otolaryngologists, and infectious disease physicians must be able to recognize and treat in a timely manner.

DIAGNOSIS AND MICROBIOLOGY

Necrotizing infections can be classified into four categories, (1) clostridial anaerobic cellulitis, (2) nonclostridial anaerobic cellulitis, (3) necrotizing fasciitis, and (4) synergistic necrotizing cellulitis.[12] In clostridial and nonclostridial anaerobic cellulitis,

[a] Department of Otolaryngology/Head and Neck Surgery, University of California Irvine School of Medicine, Orange, CA 92868, USA
[b] Department of Head and Neck Surgery, Southern California Permanente Medical Group, 3460 La Palma Avenue, Anaheim, CA 92806, USA
* Corresponding author. Department of Head and Neck Surgery, Southern California Permanente Medical Group, 3460 La Palma Avenue, Anaheim, CA 92806.
E-mail address: terryshibuya@yahoo.com

Oral Maxillofacial Surg Clin N Am 23 (2011) 425–432
doi:10.1016/j.coms.2011.04.007
1042-3699/11/$ – see front matter © 2011 Elsevier Inc. All rights reserved.

Table 1
Craniocervical necrotizing fasciitis caused by odontogenic infection

Author	Cases Reported	Years Reviewed	Cases/ Year Average
Bakshi et al,[4] 2010	7	5	1.4
Flanagan et al,[5] 2009	8	6	1.33
Sumi et al,[6] 2008	14	7	2
Kinzer et al,[7] 2009	10	8	1.25
Roccia et al,[8] 2007	9	10	0.9
Bahu et al,[1] 2001	8	10	0.8
Tung-Yiu et al,[10] 2000	11	10.5	1.05
Whitesides et al,[11] 2000	12	10	1.2
Totals	79	66.5	1.2

gas formation in the soft tissues and superficial necrosis caused by an anaerobic spore-forming and non–spore-forming organism is seen. In necrotizing fasciitis, gangrene of the skin and superficial and deep neck fascia occurs with occasional gas produced in the soft tissues by staphylococci, hemolytic streptococci, and gram-negative rods. In synergistic necrotizing cellulitis, the interaction of anaerobic and gram-negative bacteria results in myonecrosis and gas formation in the soft tissues.

Necrotizing infections have been reported to occur after massive trauma resulting in a mandible fracture or up to 3 weeks after a dental extraction.[2] Patients tend to present critically ill and often the overlying skin is discolored or gangrenous. The soft tissue of the neck to palpation demonstrates subcutaneous crepitations. Systemic symptoms include fever, toxicity, malaise, confusion, weakness, hypotension, and tachycardia. Radiologic studies reveal gas in the soft tissues of the neck or face. In addition, CT scans demonstrate obliteration between the soft tissue planes in the neck.

The microbial patterns found to cause necrotizing fasciitis are variable. The pathogens most commonly found include Group A β-hemolytic streptococci, staphylococci, and gram-negative rods. Biopsy is often the best method for obtaining cultures and sensitivities. CCNF is of polymicrobial nature, with anaerobic super infections contributing

to the myonecrosis that occurs. In the authors' experience with over 14 cases of necrotizing fasciitis in the head and neck, all of the cases have been polymicrobial, with 70% having anaerobic bacteria present.[1] The most common anaerobic bacteria isolated were Prevotella. Antibiotic coverage for CCNF organisms usually requires triple therapy. The antibiotics used must cover gram-positive, gram-negative, and anaerobic bacteria. Consultation with an infectious disease specialist is recommended. The bacteria causing CCNF grow in a synergistic fashion with the facultative anaerobes thriving on the environment created by aerobes. Once bacterial cultures and sensitivities are established, antibiotic therapy should be sensitivity directed.

ANATOMY AND PATHOPHYSIOLOGY

Dental infections can arise from pulpal and periodontally involved teeth. The degree of infection depends on the virulence of the infecting bacteria, the immune status of the patient, and the anatomy of the infected region. An infection can arise within a tooth or in the bed of an extracted tooth and may occur immediately or up to 3 weeks after extraction or treatment. For the aggressive infectious process of CCNF to occur, the infection process spreads from the tooth into the medullary space of the mandible or maxilla, then through the cortical plates of bone into the soft tissue of the face or neck. Once in the soft tissue, the infection spreads via diffuse cellulitis into a phlegmon and then into an abscess. Spread continues along the fascial planes extending along the superficial cervical neck fascia into the deep cervical neck fascia. Within the deep cervical neck fascia there are three layers: (1) superficial, (2) middle, and (3) deep. Extension of infection along these fascial planes can result in significant morbidities.

Under the epidermis and dermis of the neck lies the first layer of subcutaneous connective tissue that envelops the platysma, known as the "superficial cervical fascia." This layer contains cutaneous nerves, blood vessels, lymphatics, and varying degrees of fat deposition. The superficial cervical fascia continues on to the thorax as the platysma drapes over the clavicles on to the upper chest and shoulders. Beneath the platsyma lies the superficial layer of the deep cervical fascia. This layer of fascia, also known as the "investing fascia," surrounds the trapezious and sternocleidomastoid muscles, and the submandibular and parotid glands. In the upper neck, it extends from the anterior border of the sternocleidomastoid muscle over the mandible to the zygomatic arch superiorly and inferiorly to the hyoid bone. It is within this investing layer of fascia that it is believed CCNF spreads and must be adequately exposed and drained during the surgical approach. Deep inside of this is the middle layer of deep cervical fascia, also known as the "visceral fascia" or "pretracheal fascia."[13] This layer of fascia separates the larynx, trachea, esophagus, and thyroid gland from the surrounding structures. The middle layer of deep cervical fascia also contains the strap muscles and forms the midline raphe and the pterygomandibular raphe. Finally, the deep layer of the deep cervical fascia surrounds the vertebral column and its associated paraspinal muscles.

There are multiple fascial compartments in the neck and face where infection can spread and invade. These anatomic spaces include the canine space, buccal space, sublingual space, submandibular space, submental space, masticator space, and parapharyngeal space (**Figs. 1 and 2**).

The canine space is an area created by the quadrates labii superioris originating from the face of the maxilla. This muscle has several heads that insert on the angle of the mouth. A space exists medially between the infraorbital and zygomatic heads of this muscle and between it and the caninus muscle arising from the bone above the canine fossa. This is a region in which infection from the cuspid teeth of the maxilla can spread in a superior direction. Swelling is noted in the cheek and lateral border of the nose adjacent to the medial canthus of the eye.

The buccal space is an area created by the buccinator muscle and buccopharyngeal fascia medially, the cheek skin laterally, the lip muscles anteriorly, the pterygomandibular raphe posteriorly, the zygomatic arch superiorly, and the lower aspect of the mandible inferiorly. Infection of the maxillary and mandibular bicuspid and molar teeth through the buccal cortex can spread into this space. Swelling is noted in the cheek region, which extends medially to the middle of the upper lip, inferiorly extends to the lateral one third of the lower lip, posteriorly to the ramus and border of the parotid gland, and superiorly may entirely close the eye because of eyelid edema.

The sublingual space is an area bounded anterior and laterally by the mandible; superiorly by the floor of the mouth and tongue; inferiorly by the mylohyoid muscle; posteriorly by the hyoid bone; and medially by the genioglossus, geniohyoid, and styloglossus muscles. This space communicates freely with the opposite side of the neck and anteriorly communicates with the submental space. The mylohyoid ridge to which the muscle attaches on the inner table of the mandible slopes in a downward direction

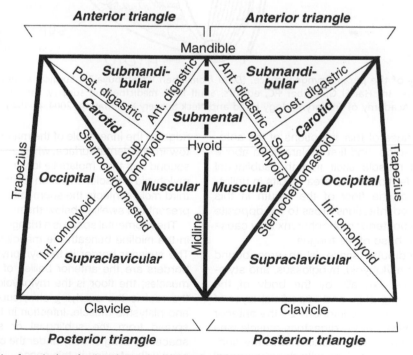

Fig. 1. Schematic of cervical neck triangles and subtriangles. (*From* Stachler RH, Shibuya TY, Golub JS, et al. General otolaryngology. In: Pasha R, editor. Otolaryngology head & neck surgery, clinical reference guide. 3rd edition. San Diego (CA): Plural Publishing Group; 2010. p. 240. Copyright © 2011 Plural Publishing, Inc. All rights reserved. Used with permission.)

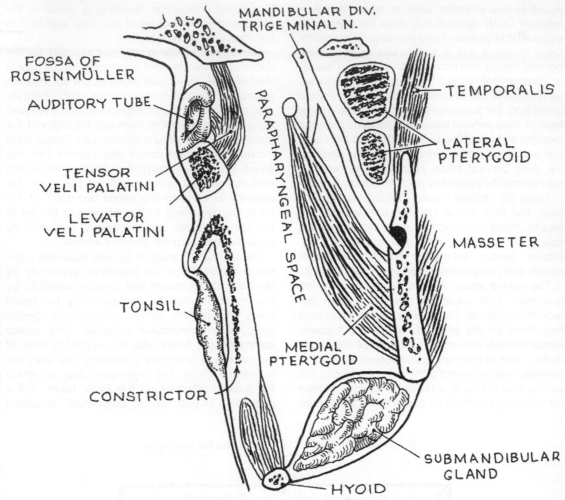

Fig. 2. Anatomy of the parapharyngeal space. (*Data from* Chen VY, Shibuya TY. Surgical anatomy of the parapharyngeal space. In: Har-El G, Weber PC, editors. Skull base medicine and surgery. 1st edition. Alexandria (VA): American Academy of Otolaryngology-Head and Neck Surgery Foundation; 2004. p. 154.)

anteriorly. Because of this, infections of the anterior teeth, bicuspids, and first molars drain above the mylohyoid muscle shelf into the sublingual space. Early infection in this area results in unilateral elevation of the floor of the mouth in this region. Advanced infections cross to the opposite side and in the posterior orphopharynx may cause elevation of the base of the tongue.

The submandibular space is an area bound medially by the mylohyoid, hyoglossus, and styloglossus muscles; laterally by the body of the mandible, overlying skin, and superficial layer of deep cervical fascia; and inferiorly by the anterior and posterior bellies of the digastrics muscle (see **Fig. 1**). It communicates anteriorly with the submental space and posteriorly with the pharyngeal space (see **Fig. 1**). Infection in this space is primarily caused by infection of the second and third molars. The mylohyoid muscle and mylohyoid

ridge on the inner table of the mandible lies higher toward the dental surface, whereas the roots of the second and third molars lie lower or inferior to the mylohyoid muscle. Infection of the second and third molars infects the submandibular space and presents as swelling below the mandible.

The submental space is a triangular area located in the midline beneath the mandible (see **Fig. 1**). The superior border is the symphysis; the lateral borders are the anterior bellies of the digastrics muscles; the floor is the mylohyoid muscle; and the roof is the overlying skin, superficial fascia, and platysma muscle. Infection in this region can spread from the sublingual or submandibular space. Swelling directly under the chin is clinically seen with infection in this space.

Ludwig angina is a term used to collectively refer to an infection that involves the submandibular, sublingual, and submental spaces. It is typically caused by infection of the mandibular molar teeth. Clinical presentation is that of brawny edema of the neck extending along the entire anterolateral neck with elevation of the floor of the mouth. As the sublingual space becomes more involved with infection, the tongue gets displaced posteriorly, resulting in airway compression.

The masticator space is divided into three compartments (masseteric, temporal, and pterygoid) and is associated with the muscle of mastication. The masseteric compartment is an area bound by the masseter muscle laterally and the ramus of the mandible medially. The pterygoid compartment is an area bound by pterygoid muscles medially and the ramus of the mandible laterally. The temporal compartment is divided into two portions. The superficial portion that lies between the superficial temporal fascia and the temporalis muscle and the deep portion that lies between the temporalis muscle and periosteum of the temporal bone. Infection in this area presents as fullness over the ramus of the mandible, fullness in the temporal region, and trismus.

The parapharyngeal space, also known as the "pharyngomaxillary space" or "lateral pharyngeal space," is an area shaped like a cone or upsidedown pyramid with its apex at the lesser cornu of the hyoid bone (see **Fig. 2**). It is bound medially by the pharynx; laterally by the ascending ramus of the mandible, pterygoid muscles, and capsule of the parotid gland; superiorly by the base of skull; inferiorly by the hyoid bone, fascia of the submandibular gland, stylohyoid muscle, and posterior belly of the digastric muscle; and posteriorly by the carotid sheath. Clinically, infection in this region presents as an intraoral bulge of the tonsil and lateral pharyngeal wall and external swelling of the soft tissues over the mandible and parotid regions (**Figs. 3** and **4**A).

The fascial layers that envelope the various structures in the neck also have varying degrees of extension into the thorax; these connections can be thought of as "superhighways" to emphasize the risk of thoracic extension. The three fascial planes that lie posterior to the aerodigestive system with connections to the thorax are as follows: (1) the retropharyngeal space, (2) the danger space, and (3) the prevertebral space. The spread of infection via the retropharyngeal space, also known as the "retrovisceral space," is found more commonly in children. This space is bound by the pharyngeal constrictor muscles anteriorly and the alar fascia posteriorly. The alar fascia is an anterior subdivision off of the prevertebral fascia that bridges between the transverse processes of the spine. The retropharyngeal

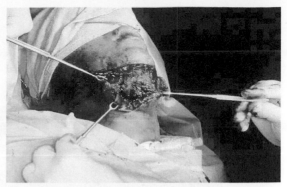

Fig. 3. Craniocervical necrotizing fasciitis presenting over the chin region with black necrosis of the underlying soft tissue.

space extends from the skull base to the arch of the aorta within the mediastinum. The danger space is located between the alar fascia and prevertebral fascia, and it extends from the skull base to the diaphragm. This space is termed the "danger space" because of its composition of loose areolar tissue and potential for rapid spread of infection. Lastly, the prevertebral space is found posterior to the prevertebral fascia, and extends from the skull base all the way to the level of the coccyx.

Anterior to the aerodigestive tract, where necrotizing fasciitis of the head and neck is most commonly found, there are essentially three different pathways of inferior spread. First, the infection could extend anterior to the sternum within the superficial cervical fascia as the platysma drapes over the clavicles onto the upper chest and shoulders. The second route, which is also the most common pathway for lethal spread of CCNF, is along the superficial layer of deep cervical fascia. This layer of fascia splits over the manubrium, and the posterior portion enters the upper mediastinum. Most commonly, the infection is contained anterior to the manubrium and exhibits subcutaneous emphysema or crepitus of the superior chest. The surgical approach does not require a sternotomy and improves prognosis significantly. The last route involves penetration of necrotizing fasciitis through the investing fascia and into the pretracheal fascia. Because the typical polymicrobial CCNF does not penetrate fascial planes, one must also consider actinomycosis in the differential diagnosis in such cases. If an aggressive infection reaches the mediastinum and internal organ damage is suspected, the prognosis becomes poor. Even if the disease process is contained within the more superficial fascial planes and reaches the chest anterior to the sternum, this can still signify an aggressive disease pattern. In the authors' experience, this has led to

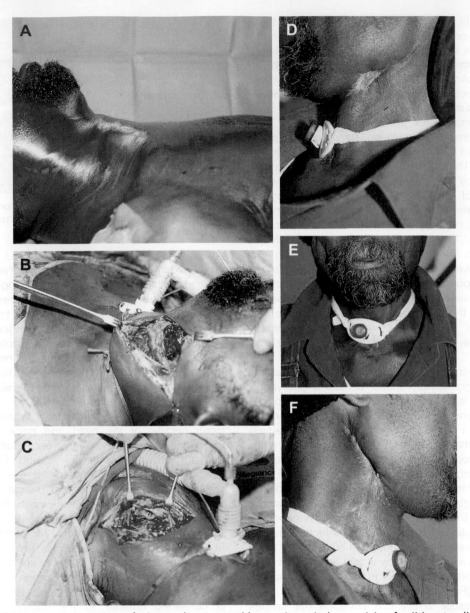

Fig. 4. (*A*) Preoperative massive soft tissue edema caused by craniocervical necrotizing fasciitis extending down the face, neck, and chest soft tissue planes. (*B*) Left neck incision exposing edematous soft tissue and necrosis. (*C*) Right neck incision exposing edematous soft tissue and necrosis. (*D*) Postoperative wound healing, view of left neck. (*E*) Midline view. (*F*) Right neck view.

a 20% increase in mortality rate once thoracic extension is present.[1]

The literature shows that CCNF complications from intrathoracic extension include mediastinitis (100%); pericarditis (12.5%); pleural effusion (12.5%); empyema (7.5%); pericardial effusion (5%); pneumonitis (5%); cardiac tamponade (2.5%); and esophageal bleed (2.5%).[3] The mortality rate from multiple case series averages around 35%.[1–11] In cases where intrathoracic

extension is suspected, a general and thoracic surgery consult is necessary. Depending on the extent of involvement, the mediastinum can be explored and debrided through a transcervical or transthoracic approach. For isolated mediastinitis, a transcervical exploration and debridement with mediastinal drain placement is often sufficient. If pleural effusion develops as a consequence of disease spread, adding chest tubes for drainage is necessary.

INCIDENCE AND FREQUENCY

The third National Health and Nutrition Examination Survey (NHANES III) found that almost 3 out of every 10 adults in the United States have untreated dental decay present. In addition, 26% of the United States population aged 20 years and older suffers from destructive periodontal disease. Although these numbers have trended downward since the prior survey (NHANES II), it still remains that 85% of adults have experienced dental caries at some point in their life.[14] Sequellae of dental infections include local and distant disease processes. Distant diseases that have been described include bacteremia, infective endocarditis, mediastinitis, and septic emboli. Local disease may be simple, such as a small periapical abscess, or extend inferiorly to involve the submandibular space and beyond. Extension through the planes of the floor of the mouth can lead to Ludwig angina, which is a potentially life-threatening disease because of its ability to compromise the airway. In this situation, the infection has reached the submandibular space; the body often encapsulates and walls-off the infection using natural barriers. However, occasionally the virulence of the bacteria can overcome the natural barriers and extend through the fascial planes to reach the neck. This is the route of spread found in most cases of CCNF. A review of the literature demonstrates that in most major metropolitan and urban medical centers, the frequency of dental infection resulting in CCNF is approximately 1.2 cases per year (see **Table 1**).

TREATMENT

CCNF requires surgical and strict medical management in addition to the triple antibiotic regimen. This antibiotic regimen provides coverage for gram-positive, gram-negative, and anaerobic bacteria. Most patients require tracheostomy tube placement at the time of neck exploration and debridement to secure and protect the patient's airway (see **Fig. 4**A–C). Because of the severity of systemic toxicity caused by CCNF, patients often suffer complications, such as acute renal failure, adult respiratory distress syndrome, pneumonia, electrolyte abnormalities, disseminated intravascular coagulopathy, seizures, sepsis, gastrointestinal bleeding, gastritis, and nephropathy. The authors typically obtain a critical care and internal medicine consultation and an infectious disease consultation. As bacterial cultures and sensitivities are obtained, antibiotics are appropriately adjusted. In addition, patients often have comorbidities, such as alcoholism, diabetes mellitus, malnutrition, or immunocompromises caused by infection or cancer.[1]

For all cases of CCNF, aggressive surgical intervention is necessary with wide incision and debridement of necrotic tissue until healthy bleeding tissue is encountered. It is typically necessary to debride necrotic muscle, fat, and salivary gland tissue. We recommend a wide incision and typically use an apron-type of incision that provides access to all zones of the neck (see **Fig. 4**B, C). Infection frequently extends inferiorly toward the mediastinum and this inferior access may be very helpful. We avoid the use of any inferior limb extending off of the neck incision because the blood supply to the skin flap is already compromised from the infection and thrombosed vessels. Once opening the neck, we carefully open all involved fascial tissue planes and compartments of the neck that are involved (submandibular, sublingual, submental, parapharyngeal, retropharyngeal, masticator, buccal, and so forth). The wound is lavaged with 3 to 5 L of saline irrigation. One instrument that is very useful for this process is the Pulsavac Plus (Zimmer, Warsaw, IN, USA), which is frequently used to irrigate and clean soft tissue and bony cavities. At the end of the procedure, the authors then place large 0.5- to 1-in Penrose drains deep into the fascial spaces and leave the wound open. This prevents infected fluid collections and allows for debridement at bedside. Repeat debridements are often necessary and should be tailored to the extent of disease and the individual response to therapy. In the authors' experience, repeated wound explorations and debridements under anesthesia facilitated wound healing and identified areas of fluid reaccumulation. They have also found that, on average, CCNF patients require three surgical debridements under general anesthesia, 11.7 days in the intensive care unit, and 24.1 days in the hospital.[1] In addition, most cases of CCNF require a tracheostomy to secure the patient's airway (see **Fig. 4**D–F).

Postoperative management of patients is done in the intensive care unit. Patients frequently require fluid resuscitation, arterial lines, and central lines. It is not uncommon for septic patients to require a vasopressor to support blood pressure.[3] In addition to daily dressing changes and repeated surgical debridements, patients may benefit from hyperbaric oxygen therapy (HBO). At the cellular level, the oxygenation enhances phagocytosis of bacteria and changes the microenvironment to an unfavorable one for anaerobic bacteria. HBO promotes angiogenesis, collagen formation, and capillary budding into the wound. In addition, improved vascularization in the wound allows for better penetration of antibiotics and leukocytes and lymphocytes into the wound bed. There is no standard HBO regimen recommended for CCNF. The authors have used a regimen of five daily dives performed at 2.4 atmospheres for 45 minutes each.

SUMMARY

CCNF is a rapidly spreading soft tissue infection of polymicrobial origin characterized by necrosis of the subcutaneous tissue and superficial fascia. Left unchecked, this infection invariably leads to systemic toxicity, multisystem organ failure, and eventual death. Complications of CCNF include airway obstruction, carotid artery occlusion, jugular vein thrombosis, mediastinitis, empyema, and pleural or pericardial effusion. In the authors' experience[1] and reports within the literature (see **Table 1**), dental infections have been found to be the leading cause of CCNF. Although it is rare to have life-threatening complications from a dentoalveolar infection, one must be aware of this disease process, understand how to diagnosis it, understand its anatomy and pathophysiology, and initiate appropriate treatment in a timely manner.

REFERENCES

1. Bahu SJ, Shibuya TY, Meleca RJ, et al. Craniocervical necrotizing fasciitis: an 11-year experience. Otolaryngol Head Neck Surg 2001;125:245–52.
2. Levine TM, Wurster CF, Krepsi YP. Mediastinitis occurring as a complication of odontogenic infection. Laryngoscope 1986;96:747–50.
3. Lalwani AK, Kaplan MJ. Mediastinal and thoracic complications of necrotizing fasciitis of the head and neck. Head Neck 1991;13:531–9.
4. Bakshi J, Virk RS, Jain A, et al. Cervical necrotizing fasciitis: our experience with 11 cases and our technique for surgical debridement. Ear Nose Throat J 2010;89(2):84–6.
5. Flanagan CE, Daramola OO, Maisel RH, et al. Surgical debridement and adjunctive hyperbaric oxygen in cervical necrotizing fasciitis. Otolaryngol Head Neck Surg 2009;140(5):730–4.
6. Sumi Y, Ogura H, Nakamori Y, et al. Nonoperative catheter management for cervical necrotizing fasciitis with and without descending necrotizing mediastinitis. Arch Otolaryngol Head Neck Surg 2008;134(7):750–6.
7. Kinzer S, Pfeiffer J, Becker S, et al. Severe deep neck space infections and mediastinitis of odontogenic origin: clinical relevance and implications for diagnosis and treatment. Acta Otolaryngol 2009;129(1):62–70.
8. Roccia F, Pecorari GC, Oliaro A, et al. Ten years of descending necrotizing mediastinitis: management of 23 cases. J Oral Maxillofac Surg 2007;65(9):1716–24.
9. Umeda M, Minamikawa T, Komatsubara H, et al. Necrotizing fasciitis caused by dental infection: a retrospective analysis of 9 cases and a review of the literature. Oral Surg Oral Med Oral Pathol Oral Radiol Endod 2003;95(3):283–90.
10. Tung-Yiu W, Jehn-Shyun H, Ching-Hung C, et al. Cervical necrotizing fasciitis of odontogenic origin: a report of 11 cases. J Oral Maxillofac Surg 2000;58(12):1347–52.
11. Whitesides L, Cotto-Cumba C, Myers RA. Cervical necrotizing fasciitis of odontogenic origin: a case report and review of 12 cases. J Oral Maxillofac Surg 2000;58(2):144–51.
12. Lawson W, Reino AJ, Westreich RW. Odontogenic infections. In: Bailey BJ, Johnson JT, editors. Head & neck surgery: otolaryngology. Philadelphia (PA): Lippincott Williams and Wilkins; 2006. p. 615–30.
13. Agur DMR. Grant's atlas of anatomy. 12th edition. Philadelphia (PA): Lippincott Williams and Wilkins; 2007.
14. CDC. Third National Health and Nutrition Examination Survey (NHANES III) 1988–1994. Atlanta (GA): National Center for Health Statistics, Centers for Disease Control and Prevention; 1994.

Complications in Bone Grafting

Alan S. Herford, DDS, MD*, Jeffrey S. Dean, DDS, MD

KEYWORDS
- Bone grafts • Autogenous grafts • Bone harvest
- Graft complications

Bone grafts are often necessary to restore missing tissue and to provide structural support for implants. Alveolar bone remodeling/resorption after tooth extraction can make it difficult to place implants in adequate bone. This can result in a poor aesthetic outcome and possible premature loss of the implants.[1,2] The need for maxillary and mandibular bone grafting is often necessary to provide adequate bone for implant placement. Various types of grafting material can be used to augment the deficient alveolus, including the use of autogenous bone. Autogenous grafts remain the gold standard because of their osteogenic properties and because they are more predictable than allografts or xenografts, especially for larger defects.

The uses of cortical and cancellous bone have different indications and require a thorough understanding of what the indications are for each. Bone heals by cellular regeneration and it is this cellular regeneration that allows bone grafts to form bone rather than forming scar. The osteogenic properties of autogenous bone make it an ideal choice for bone grafting and is more predictable when grafting large defects. Selecting an augmentation material for grafting requires knowledge of the material being used with regards to biocompatibility, bioresorbability, structural stability, availability, ease of handling, and costs.

With the biologic and technical demands associated with bone grafting, various complications can occur. It is important to understand and manage complications associated with bone grafting to minimize poor outcomes and failure. Complications may result from the harvesting of the bone graft or may develop secondarily at the grafted site. Donor site complications include damage to local anatomic structures—teeth, nerves, muscles, vasculature, and infection (iliac crest bone graft complications have been as high as 15%–25%)—and the recipient site with possible complications of sinus disease, early or delayed exposure of the graft, or resorption of the graft and infection.[3–6] Complications associated at the grafted site may lead to larger defects with loss of bone volume and soft tissue defects. Further interventions to correct the problem (additional grafting with associated donor site morbidity) may be necessary.

BIOLOGY OF BONE FORMATION

The biology of bone formation involves osteogenesis, osteoconduction, and osteoinduction. Osteoprogenitor cells found within bone are stem cell precursors that can differentiate into various connective tissue lines. Corticocancellous block bone is still a viable choice in grafting and is used successfully. Cancellous bone, considered the gold standard in grafting, provides the greatest amount of osteoprogenitor cells and allows for rapid vascularization. Bone morphogenic proteins are released from the mineral matrix in bone to induce stem cells within the graft to form mature bone.[7]

HARVEST SITES

Many sites are available for graft harvest, including local and distant sites (**Table 1**). Consideration as

Department of Oral and Maxillofacial Surgery, Loma Linda University, 11092 Anderson Street, Loma Linda, CA 92350, USA
* Corresponding author. Department of Oral and Maxillofacial Surgery, Loma Linda University School of Dentistry, Room 3306, 11092 Anderson Street, Loma Linda CA 92350.
E-mail address: aherford@llu.edu

Oral Maxillofacial Surg Clin N Am 23 (2011) 433–442
doi:10.1016/j.coms.2011.04.004

Table 1
Harvest sites

Donor Site	Type of Graft	Volume Available	Possible Complications
Ascending Ramus	Cortical	5–10 cc	Damage to the neurovascular bundle with resulting temporary or permanent neurosensory disturbance
Symphysis	Corticocancellous	5–10 cc	Ectropion of the lower lip and chin ptosis Damage to the teeth and mental nerve with neurosensory disturbance
Tuberosity	Cancellous	2 cc	Oroantral communication
Tibia	Cancellous	20–40 cc	Tibial plateau fracture Interference with growth plate in children
Cranium	Cortical	20–40 cc	Damage to dura and brain
Anterior Iliac Crest	Corticocancellous	50–70 cc	Gait disturbance Paresthesia of the lateral thigh Hernia Hematoma
Posterior Iliac Crest	Corticocancellous	80–140 cc	Gait disturbance Paresthesia of the posterior regions Hematoma

to which site is used depends on the size and geometry of the defect. The quantity and quality of the bone needed are important when choosing a donor site. The technique chosen for grafting (particulate or block) also helps determines the preferred donor site.

Local Sites for Bone Harvesting

Bone harvested from local sites has advantages over other more distant donor sites (**Fig. 1**). The proximity of the graft is of convenience and

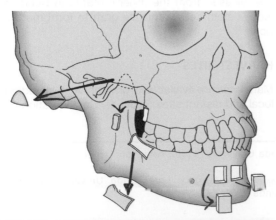

Fig. 1. Local sites commonly used for harvest of grafts.

eliminates the possible complications from an extraoral site, such as scarring, gait disturbance, or need for hospitalization. The grafts also provide bone with similar architecture as the bone at the recipient site. A disadvantage is the limited amount of bone available compared with other extraoral sites.

Maxillary tuberosity

Bone harvested from the maxillary tuberosity has limited use as a donor graft because of the small volume available. The graft material is cancellous and can be harvested with simultaneous third molar removal. Complications associated with this site include oral/antral communication and hematoma formation from disruption pterygoid venous plexus.

Ascending ramus

The anterior portion of the ascending ramus has been used for grafting in a variety of clinical applications (**Fig. 2**). Bone harvested from the ascending ramus provides mainly a cortical graft with a volume of approximately 5 to 10 cc. The bone obtained from the ramus is a good option for horizontal defects requiring onlay grafting. These grafts heal quickly, exhibit minimal resorption, and maintain their dense quality. Possible complications of mandibular ramus graft site include damage to

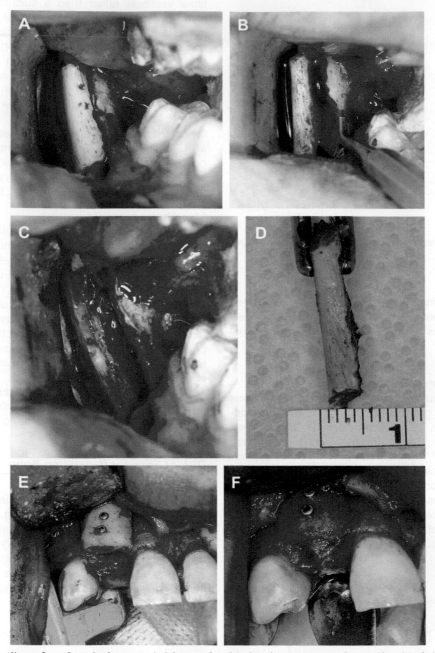

Fig. 2. (*A*) Outline of graft to be harvested. (*B*) Use of a chisel to harvest ramus bone. The chisel should not be directed toward the neurovascular bundle. (*C*) The uninjured neurovascular bundle is visualized after harvest of the graft. (*D*) Thickness of the graft. (*E*) Bone graft secured into place with screws. (*F*) Bone graft is well integrated with surrounding bone.

the neurovascular bundle with neurosensory disturbance, infection, damage to tooth roots if extending into an area of molar teeth, and trismus. The lingual nerve is also at risk during harvest from the ramus, either due to poor incision placement, aggressive retraction of a lingual flap, or

damage during suturing. Misch[8] compared intraoral donor sites for onlay grafting before implant placement and found that the ramus was associated with fewer complications than the symphysis graft as a donor site (**Fig. 3**). Silva and colleagues[9] found that 8.3% of patients who had had bone

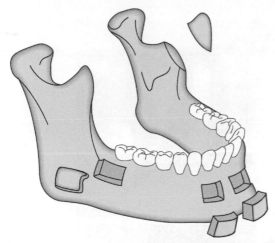

Fig. 3. Harvest area of the ramus and symphysis region.

harvested from the mandibular ramus reported a sensory deficit whereas 16% of patients undergoing harvest from the symphysis had a sensory deficit.

Mandibular symphysis

The mandibular symphysis allows ease of access to bone for grafting, good bone quality for localized repair, a corticocancellous block graft morphology, and minimal graft resorption (**Fig. 4**).[10,11] The graft can provide either a block or particulate graft material. Bone harvested contains more cancellous bone than other intraoral sites, thus providing a greater amount of osteoprogenitor cells. The lower lip/soft tissue chin may become ptotic after surgery in this area with poor mentalis muscle suspension.[12] Incision in the

labial vestibule rather than a sulcular approach allows preservation of the crestal bone and allows a more secure closure with reapproximation of the mentalis muscle, resulting in less risk of chin ptosis. Clavero and Lundgren[13] compared symphysis and ramus harvest sites and reported a higher rate of altered sensation in patients in whom bone was harvested from the symphysis. In their series of patients, 52% of patients (symphysis) still had some decreased sensitivity at 18 months after surgery. Patients who had bone harvested from the ramus had what was considered a permanent nerve injury. Infections are minimal for these harvest sites (<1%).[14]

Mandibular coronoid process

Bone harvested from the mandibular coronoid process is primarily cortical bone similar to calvarial bone and can be used for up to 1-tooth and 2-tooth sites. The harvest can extend up to 5 mm below the sigmoid notch so as to not interfere with the inferior alveolar neurovascular bundle.[5] Harvesting the bone is relatively easy and done through an intraoral approach dissecting the temporalis from its attachment. A side cutting bur or reciprocating saw is used to perform an osteotomy of the coronoid process.

Advantages of this harvest site include no facial scarring or damage to teeth. Possible complications include trismus or damage to the buccal branch of the trigeminal nerve.

Distant Sites for Harvesting Bone

Calvarial bone

Calvarial bone can be used for facial, maxillary, and mandibular reconstruction (**Fig. 5**). It was described as an autogenous bone graft by Tessier in 1982.[15] Calvarial bone is mainly cortical in nature and generally used for onlay grafting. Harvesting calvarial bone is relatively easy and safe. Partial-thickness and full-thickness calvarial grafts

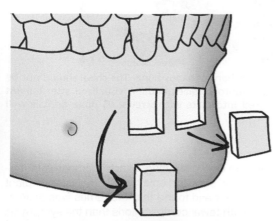

Fig. 4. Harvest of corticocancellous graft from the symphyseal region.

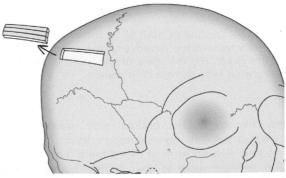

Fig. 5. Harvest of a monocortical calvarial graft from the parietal bone.

can be used. The skull has 3 layers the outer cortex, medullary space (diploe), and an inner cortex. Gonzalez and colleagues[16] found that the average thickness of the skull was 6.3 mm with a range of 5.3 to 7.5 mm. The posterior parietal bone having the greatest thickness and is the preferred site for harvesting bone for grafting. The harvest site is covered by tissue that is usually hair bearing, which camouflages scarring.

Complications associated with harvesting calvarial bone include the possibility of dural tear, epidural hematoma, alopecia, hematoma, infection, contour deformity, and scarring with alopecia the most common complication.

Tibial bone

Catone and colleagues[17] described the proximal tibia as a source for cancellous bone used in maxillary reconstruction in 1992. It is relatively easy to harvest and can be done in the office as outpatient surgery (**Fig. 6**). The volume of available cancellous bone harvested from the proximal tibia can be up to 40 cc. The lateral approach to the tibia for cancellous bone is over Gerdy tubercle. Gerdy tubercle is easily palpated, located between the tibial tuberosity and the fibular head and has no vital structures overlying it. A medial approach has also been described. Herford and colleagues[18] compared the medial with the lateral approach and found no statistical difference in the

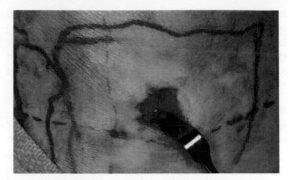

Fig. 7. Harvest of bone from a medial approach.

mean volume of bone harvested from either site (**Fig. 7**). They also reported that the bone is closer to the skin and is more distant to vital structures compared with the lateral approach.

The incidence of complications for tibial bone harvest ranges from 1.3% to 3.8%, which compares favorably with the 8.6% to 9.2% incidence of complications associated with harvest of iliac crest bone.[17,18] Complications associated with tibial bone harvest may include prolonged pain, gait disturbance, wound dehiscence, osteomyelitis, wound infection, hematoma, seroma, paresthesia, fracture, and violation of the joint space. No tibial fractures have been reported. The risks of this procedure need to be discussed with patients and, because gait disturbances

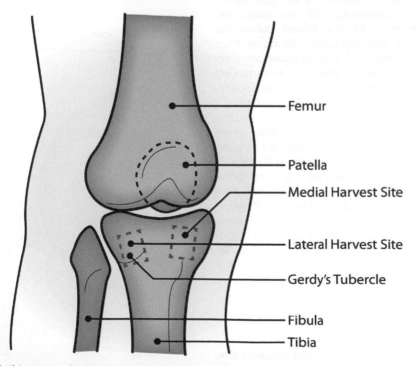

Femur

Patella

Medial Harvest Site

Lateral Harvest Site

Gerdy's Tubercle

Fibula

Tibia

Fig. 6. Proximal tibia anatomic structures.

have been reported, patients should be consented appropriately. Contraindications for harvesting bone from the tibia include the need for a block graft, growing patients, patients with a history of knee injury or surgery, or patients with advanced arthritic disease.

Iliac crest bone

Bone harvested from the anterior or posterior pelvis can provide a great quantity of grafting material. The anterior iliac crest is a good source of cortical and cancellous bone for grafting. Up to 50 cc of cancellous bone can be harvested from the anterior iliac crest. This approach can be done in the operating room or in the ambulatory setting. The bone is harvested with or without a cortical segment. The incision is made approximately 1 cm posterior to the anterior superior iliac spine and is carried down to the crest of the ilium. The skin is retracted medially to keep the incision from lying directly over the crest, thus preventing irritation from clothing resting on the incision.

Complications associated with iliac crest bone grafts range from 0.76% to 25% (major) and 9.4% to 24% (minor).[19] These include bleeding, hematoma, perforation of the bowel, hernia, ileus, pain, gait disturbance, cosmetic deformity, injury to sensory nerves, and infection. Fractures of the iliac crest can also be seen and are treated conservatively.[20] Care must also be taken to avoid injury to the sensory nerves (**Fig. 8**). The nerves that may be injured include the iliohypogastric, lateral femoral cutaneous, and the subcostal, which is a branch of the lateral cutaneous nerve.[21–23] Joshi and Kostakis[24] found in their series of 114 patients that 10% experienced pain for greater than 16 weeks and 23% experienced some difficulty in ambulation 6 weeks postoperatively. In a prospective study by Rudman,[25] patients did not have delayed ambulation or prolonged hospitalization. These patients were treated for alveolar clefts and represented a young patient population. Ahlmann and colleagues[26] compared anterior and posterior iliac crest bone harvests in terms of harvest site morbidity. This study involved 88 consecutive patients (108 grafting procedures). The anterior approach was associated with more complications than the posterior approach, 8% versus 2%, respectively (**Fig. 9**). Postoperative pain was significantly of greater duration after anterior harvests.

COMPLICATIONS ASSOCIATED WITH THE GRAFTED SITE

Complications can also occur at the recipient site. Possible complications include loosening and/or

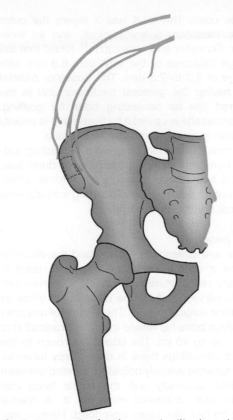

Fig. 8. Harvest site for the anterior iliac bone harvest.

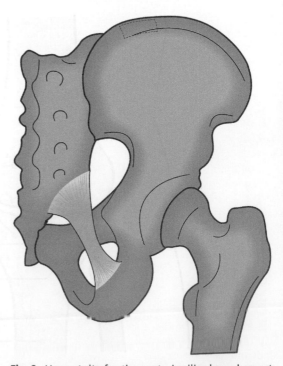

Fig. 9. Harvest site for the posterior iliac bone harvest.

resorption of the graft, localized infection, or damage to adjacent anatomic structures, such as the neurovascular bundle.[27] Damage to adjacent teeth and complete loss of the graft are also possibilities. Even with tension-free closure, a significant amount of exposures of the underlying graft occurs (**Figs. 10–13**). The earlier the occurrence after placement of the graft, the more likely loss of the entire graft may occur.[28] Membranes (resorbable and nonresorbable) may be placed to thicken the tissue over the graft and prevent or at least delay exposure of the graft. Membranes are routinely used as a part of the guided bone regeneration technique and aid in preventing competing, nonosteogenic tissue from infiltrating the grafted bone.

A study by Louis and colleagues[29] recently evaluated patients who received mandibular or maxillary reconstruction with autogenous particulate bone graft and titanium mesh for the purpose of implant placement. The mean augmentation for all sites was 13.7 mm (12.8 mm in the maxilla and 13.9 mm in the mandible). Totals of 82 implants were placed in the maxilla and 92 implants were placed in the mandible. In the maxillary group, 7 (55%) sites had exposure of the titanium mesh and 16 (36%) sites were exposed in the mandible (52% total). The success of the bone grafting procedure was 97.72%. They concluded that titanium mesh is a reliable containment system for grafting and the mesh tolerates exposure very well and gives predictable results.

The use of membranes may also contribute to complications. Chaushu and colleagues[30] reported soft tissue complications, including membrane exposure (42 [30.7%] of 137); incision line opening (41 [30%] of 137); and perforation of the mucosa over the grafted bone (19 [14%] of 137). Infection of the grafted site occurred in 18 (13%) of 137 bone grafts. Alveolar ridge deficiency location had a statistically significant effect on the outcome of recipient site complications. More complications were noted in the mandible compared with the maxilla. Age and gender had no statistically significant effect. Gielkens and colleagues[31] performed a meta-analysis to evaluate the available evidence that barrier membranes prevent bone resorption in autologous onlay bone grafts. The primary outcome measure was bone resorption. The search yielded 182 articles. Although most investigators concluded that they had found evidence for the protective effect of barrier membrane on bone resorption in bone grafts, the systematic review reveals that the available evidence is too weak to support this. Most of the included studies were animal experiments; thus, extrapolation to the human situation

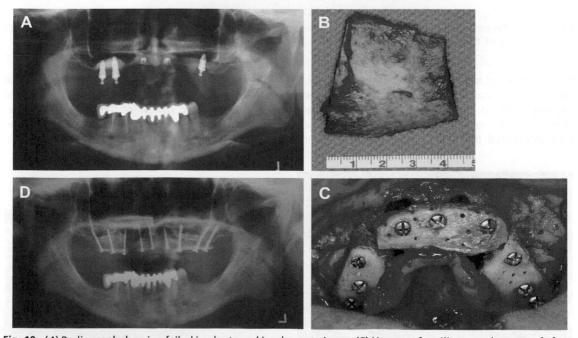

Fig. 10. (A) Radiograph showing failed implants and inadequate bone. (B) Harvest of an iliac crest bone graft from and anterior approach. (C) The grafts are secured with screws to prevent mobility of the graft. (D) Radiograph showing the grafted bone in place.

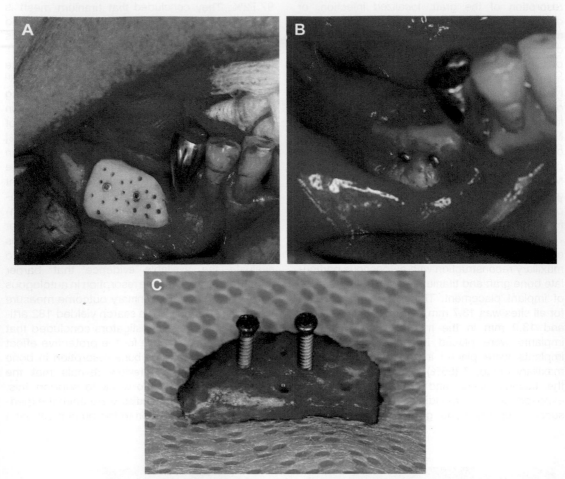

Fig. 11. (*A*) Placement of graft harvested from the ascending ramus. (*B*) Exposure of the graft postoperatively. (*C*) Complete loss of the graft.

is difficult. Most studies also had a small number of test sites, and sample size justification was generally not reported. Furthermore, ambiguity and lack of significance were found in many studies along with additional limitations, such as implantation site, unsuitable designs, and varying outcome measures. Gielkens and colleagues felt that based on a systematic review of the literature, further evidence was needed to determine whether barrier membranes prevent bone resorption in autologous onlay bone grafts.

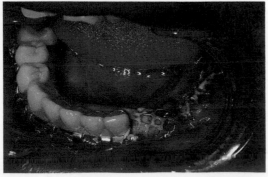

Fig. 12. Exposure of a titanium mesh within 1 week postoperatively.

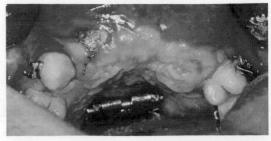

Fig. 13. Exposure of the titanium mesh months after surgery.

SUMMARY

Autogenous bone grafts continue to have wide use for reconstructing alveolar defects because of the many advantages associated with them. Although complications are low, the harvest of bone grafts does have the risk of morbidity, which varies based on the harvest site chosen. Patients should be informed of possible complications associated with bone harvest as well as complications that many develop at the grafted site.

REFERENCES

1. Herford AS, Brown BR. Outpatient harvest of bone grafts. Selected Readings in Oral and Maxillofacial Surgery 2007;15:1–14.
2. Zouhary KJ. Bone graft harvesting from distant sites: concepts and techniques. Oral Maxillofac Surg Clin North Am 2010;22:301–16.
3. Raghoebar GM, Louwerse C, Kalk WW, et al. Morbidity of chin bone harvesting. Clin Oral Implants Res 2001;12:503–7.
4. Beirne JC, Barry HJ, Brady FA, et al. Donor site morbidity of the anterior iliac crest following cancellous bone harvest. Int J Oral Maxillofac Surg 1996; 25:268–71.
5. Sittitavornwong S, Rajesh G. Bone graft harvesting from regional sites. Oral Maxillofac Surg Clin North Am 2010;22:317–30.
6. Larson PE. Morbidity associated with calvarial bone graft harvest. J Oral Maxillofac Surg 1989;47(8): 110–1.
7. Marx R. Bone and bone graft healing. Oral Maxillofac Surg Clin North Am 2007;19:455–66.
8. Misch CM. Comparison of intraoral donor site for onlay grafting prior to implant placement. Int J Oral Maxillofac Implants 1997;12:767–76.
9. Silva FM, Cortez AL, Morekira RW, et al. Complications of intraoral donor site for bone grafting prior to implant placement. Implant Dent 2006;15:420–6.
10. Gapski R, Wang HL, Misch CE. Management of incision design in symphysis graft procedures: a review of the literature. J Oral Implantol 2001;27: 134–42.
11. Weibull L, Widmark G, Ivanoff CJ, et al. Morbidity after chin bone harvesting—a retrospective long-term follow-up study. Clin Implant Dent Relat Res 2009;11:149–57.
12. Chaushu G, Blinder D, Taicher S, et al. The effect of precise reattachment of the mentalis muscle on the soft tissue response to genioplasty. J Oral Maxillofac Surg 2001;59:510–6.
13. Calvero J, Lundgren S. Ramus or chin grafts for maxillary sinus inlay and local onlay augmentation: comparison of donor site morbidity and complications. Clin Implant Dent Relat Res 2003; 5(3):154–60.
14. Pikos M. Mandibular block autografts for alveolar ridge augmentation. Atlas Oral Maxillofac Surg Clin North Am 2005;13:91–107.
15. Tessier P. Autogenous bone grafts taken from the calvarium for facial and cranial applications. Clin Plast Surg 1982;9:531–8.
16. Gonzalez AM, Papay FE, Zin JE. Calvarial thickness and its relation to cranial bone harvest. Plast Reconstr Surg 2006;117(6):1964–71.
17. Catone GA, Reimer BL, McNeir D, et al. Tibia-autogenous cancellous bone as an alternative donor site in maxillofacial surgery: a preliminary report. J Oral Maxillofac Surg 1992;50:1256–63.
18. Herford AS, King BJ, Audia F, et al. Medial approach for tibial bone graft: anatomic study and clinical technique. J Oral Maxillofac Surg 2003;61: 358–63.
19. Fowler BL, Dall BE, Rowe DE. Complications associated with harvesting autogneous iliac bone graft. Am J Orthop 1995;24:895–903.
20. Arribas-Garcia I, Alcala-Galiano A, Garcia AF, et al. Fracture of the anterior iliac crest following monocortical bone graft harvest in bisphosphonate-related mandibular pathological fracture: a case report. Oral Surg Oral Med Oral Pathol Oral Radiol Endod 2009;107:e12–4.
21. Banwart JC, Asher MA, Hassanein RS. Iliac crest bone graft donor site morbidity. A statistical evaluation. Spine 1995;20:1055–60.
22. Seiler JG 3rd, Johnson J. Iliac crest atogenous bone grafting: donor site complications. J South Orthop Assoc 2000;9:91–7.
23. Chou D, Storm PB, Campbell JN. Vulnerability of the subcostal nerve to injury during bone graft harvesting from the iliac crest. J Neurosurg 2004;1:87–9.
24. Joshi A, Kostakis GC. An investigation of postoperative morbidity following iliac crest graft harvesting. Br Dent J 2004;196:167.
25. Rudman RA. Prospective evaluation of morbidity associated with iliac crest harvest for alveolar grafting. J Oral Maxillofac Surg 1997;55:219.
26. Ahlmann E, Patzakis M, Roidis N, et al. Comparison of anterior and posterior iliac crest bone grafts in terms of harvest-site morbidity and functional outcomes. J Bone Joint Surg Am 2002;84:716.
27. Rabelo GD, de Paula PM, Rocha FS, et al. Retrospective study of bone grafting procedures before implant placement. Implant Dent 2010;19:342–50.
28. Roccuzzo M, Ramieri G, Bunino M, et al. Autogenous bone graft alone or assoiated with titanium mesh or vertical alveolar ridge augmentation: a controlled clinical trial. Clin Oral Implants Res 2007;18:286–94.
29. Louis PJ, Gutta R, Said-Al-Naief N. Reconstruction of the maxilla and mandible with particulate bone

graft and titanium mesh for implant placement. J Oral Maxillofac Surg 2008;66(2):235–45.

30. Chaushu G, Mardinger O, Peleg M. Analysis of complications following augmentation with cancellous block allografts. J Periodontol 2010;81(12):1759–64.

31. Gielkens PF, Bos RR, Raghoebar GM. Is there evidence that barrier membranes prevent bone resorption in autologous bone grafts during the healing period? A systematic review. Int J Oral Maxillofac Implants 2007;22(3):390–8.

Bisphosphonates and Oral Health: Primer and an Update for the Practicing Surgeon

Leon A. Assael, DMD

KEYWORDS

• Bisphosphonates • Oral health osteoporosis
• Bone metabolism

Oral and intravenous bisphosphonates have been in clinical use for two decades for the treatment of patients with malignancy, osteoporosis, and other diseases affecting bone metabolism. The purpose of this article is to review the features of these drugs, their effect on the diseases they treat, the oral findings associated with their use, and the assessment of osteonecrosis incidence, and pathophysiology, with some insights into treatment.

DRUG THERAPEUTIC ACTION

The mechanism of action of all bisphosphonates is delivery to the target tissue either from, in the case of oral bisphosphonates, the gut, where approximately 1% is absorbed, or via direct intravenous infusion. Once delivered, high concentrations of these drugs are observed in the developing hydroxyapatite matrix where fresh osteoid is being laid down in bone and in the kidneys. In the bone, bisphosphonates are ingested by active osteoclasts that break down the hydroxyapatite matrix and, to some extent, by osteoblasts. Other cells are also affected by administration of bisphosphonates and this might be important in understanding their effects. At high doses, there is an antiangiogenic and antitumor effect.[1] Bisphosphonates also have a less-understood influence on nutrition and communication among osteocytes, an inhibitory effect on osteoblasts, and effects on epithelium and other cells.[2]

The therapeutic action of bisphosphonates is in great part, as understood to date, to inhibit the function of osteoclasts through disruption of their cellular enzymatic activities (farnesyl disphosphate synthase associated with prenylation) that lead to bone resorption and, by inducing osteoclast apoptosis, resulting in a severe reduction in the number of osteoclasts. Loss of function of osteoclasts exposed to bisphosphonates is demonstrated by the loss of ruffled layer, demonstrating inactivation of the osteoclast or by cell death. Drops in population of osteoclasts in patients taking intravenous bisphosphonates are in excess of 95%, and these drops are persistent long after withdrawal of medication.

This reduction of activity and number of osteoclasts profoundly inhibits bone resorption, which is the primary therapeutic effect of bisphosphonates. In patients with malignancy, this can reduce the destruction of bone associated with bone metastases and thus inhibit the growth of the malignancy in bone. Malignancy metastatic to bone requires the development of an ecologic niche for the tumor, including space, blood supply, and oxygen. Tumors in bone produce parathormone–like substances that activate osteoclasts to help create this environment. Thus, active osteoclasts are the abettors of tumor growth in bone. When the intravenous bisphosphonate is used, far fewer osteoclasts are available to be recruited and the growth of the bone metastasis is inhibited. Mitigating the active focal destruction of bone by tumors also decreases the risk of pathologic fracture at the site of actively growing tumor as well as at other sites

Oral and Maxillofacial Surgery, School of Dentistry, School of Medicine, Hospital Dentistry, Oregon Health and Science University, 611 South West Campus Drive, SDOMS, Portland, OR 97239, USA
E-mail address: assael@ohsu.edu

Oral Maxillofacial Surg Clin N Am 23 (2011) 443–453
doi:10.1016/j.coms.2011.04.002
1042-3699/11/$ – see front matter © 2011 Published by Elsevier Inc.

affected by the pseudohyperparathyroidism of malignancy, produced by the systemic release of parathormone-like tumor products.

By increasing the bone mineral levels in patients with bone metastases, patients are less prone to skeletal-related events (SREs), such as pathologic fracture of long bone and rib, and compression fractures of the spine that can result in paralysis. SREs are associated with loss of function, need for extended care facilities, and shorter survival. In addition, inhibiting osteoclast function can mitigate hypercalcemia of malignancy and extend life in those patients through mitigation of the cardiac effect of hypercalcemia. Despite all these presumed positive metabolic effects of bisphosphonates, debate continues as to whether adjunctive use of bisphosphonates with other cancer therapy extends life in aggregate populations of cancer patients, with tumor-dependent conflicting data on this subject.

For patients with osteoporosis, the risk of fracture can be devastating. Approximately 3 million osteoporotic fractures occur annually in the United States, of which 300,000 are devastating hip fractures.[3] Patients with hip fractures in particular suffer from a loss of autonomy, undergo extensive rehabilitation, and are often unable to return to activities of daily living. Approximately 1 in 6 patients with osteoporotic hip fracture die in the year after that injury from a variety of related and unrelated causes.

Far less potent bisphosphonates with less-effective dose (reduced by, on average, 10 to 1 compared with intravenous bisphosphonates) are intentionally used for osteoporosis. Unlike the severe reductions in osteoclast populations with intravenous bisphosphonate use, oral bisphosphonates are designed to tip the balance with each bone remodeling cycle toward greater apposition of bone compared with loss. Hence, years of administration are required to offer any increase in bone mineral density (BMD) or lowering of fracture risk. Many studies use 3 years of oral administration to develop comparisons between those patients given a bisphosphonate and a placebo group. Reductions in osteoporotic fractures over those periods are between 40% and 70%, depending on site of fracture.[4]

Although those findings are compelling, less is known about the long-term effectiveness of bisphosphonates. The main surrogate for understanding decreased fracture risk in patients exposed to bisphosphonates is the increased BMD associated with use. As each bone remodeling cycle is completed, less of the existing hydroxyapatite/type I collagen matrix is removed. Concern in recent years regarding the effectiveness of this bone in resisting fracture has been raised as this denser, but less remodeled, bone ages. In the clinical setting, subtrocanter fractures of the femur of a spiral nature are reported that are less amenable to reduction and fixation in patients with long-term bisphosphonate use.[5] Although an increase in BMD is needed in osteoporosis, the character and vitality of the bisphosphonate exposed bone in the long-term remains an open question. The aging of collagen excreted by patients with long-standing bisphosphonate use might indicate how bones with a higher BMD could be getting weaker.[6] Older collagen submitting to the bone remodeling cycle is not likely to undergo as effective as younger collagen remodeling. This may demonstrate long-term changes in patients exposed to bisphosphonates that differ from the early changes reported in 3-year studies.

HISTORY

Bisphosphonates (previously known as diphosphonates) were first synthesized in the nineteenth century and are simple molecules with a carbon atom at the center and 2 phosphate molecules attached on either side.[7] Also attached to the other 2 carbon sites are the R1 and R2 sites completing the 4 typical attachments to the un-ionized carbon atom (**Fig. 1**). The R2 site is where nearly all of the differences among bisphosphonate pharmacology occur. R2 site are either nitrogen containing or non-nitrogen containing.

The R1 site is always a OH⁻ (hydroxide) or, in the case of clodronate, a non-nitrogen bisphosphonate (in use for osteoporosis in Europe but not the United States); both R1 and R2 sites are Cl⁻ (chloride) attachments. All bisphosphonates available as Food and Drug Administration–approved

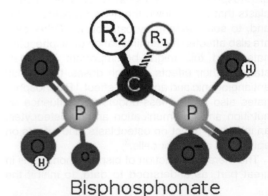

Bisphosphonate

Fig. 1. Skeleton of the bisphosphonate molecule. R2 site is the principle location of alteration for pharmacologic purposes in nitrogen bisphosphonates. (*Courtesy of* Michael David Jones, Vancouver, British Columbia, Canada.)

drugs in the United States are nitrogen-containing bisphosphonates designed for oral or intravenous administration.

The first oral bisphosphonate in the United States, alendronate (Fosamax, Merck) was introduced in the 1990s for the treatment of postmenopausal osteoporosis to reduce the risk of fractures, especially of the hip, spine, and extremities. Newer oral bisphosphonates differ only in the R2 site nitrogen side chain, including risendronate (Actonel, Procter & Gamble), for the treatment of postmenopausal osteoporosis and corticosteroid-induced osteoporosis,[8] and ibandronate (Boniva, Roche) for treatment of postmenopausal osteoporosis.[9] In addition to postmenopausal osteoporosis, oral bisphosphonates are in a large clinical trial for male osteoporosis and steroid-induced osteoporosis.[10] Anecdotal use of oral bisphosphonates for Paget disease, osteodystrophy of renal failure, and hyperparathyroidism as well as giant cell lesions are reported.

Intravenous bisphosphonates were developed for infusion, usually once monthly for patients with cancer metastatic to bone. They were designed for this use due to their ability to increase BMD and to suppress osteoclasts that are the responders to the release of parathormone-like substances by tumors in bone, which allows for the ecologic niche of tumors in bone.

FREQUENCY OF USE

Of the approximately 250,000 Americans with metastatic bone cancer at any given time, approximately half take intravenous bisphosphonate, either pamidronate (Aredia) or zoledronate (Zometa), usually once monthly. The greatest number of these patients have metastatic breast cancer with somewhat fewer having myeloma, prostate cancer, lung cancer, or renal cell carcinoma. Recently, zoledronate has been studied for the prevention/delay of bone metastases in patients with breast cancer.[11]

To date, hundreds of millions of prescriptions worldwide have been given for oral bisphosphonates for the treatment of osteoporosis.[12] Patient compliance with use can be compromised due to the side effects of administration and the infrequency of dosing. Thus, intravenous bisphosphonates are now used once quarterly, in the case of ibandronate, or once yearly, in the case of zoledronate for the treatment of osteoporosis.

Intravenous bisphosphonates are used for osteoporosis not only because of patient compliance issues but also due to the effects of oral bisphosphonates on causing esophageal inflammation and

possible severe gastrointestinal sequelae if administration by mouth does not cease. At the same time, intravenous bisphosphonates, alternatively, are associated with a flu-like syndrome after administration, sometimes effectively treated with nonsteroidal anti-inflammatory drugs, and with bone pain after administration.

GENERAL CRANIOMAXILLOFACIAL EFFECTS OF BISPHOSPHONATES

In all reports on bisphosphonates until 2003, focus was on the effect on alveolar bone health and periodontal disease was emphasized. For example, there were reports of improved outcome of periodontal disease in women taking bisphosphonates.[13] Imaging findings of the dentoalveolar region demonstrated increase BMD, but maxillofacial skeleton were not observed at that time nor was osteonecrosis. The only complications of the oral and maxillofacial region were headache and myofascial pain.

A placebo-controlled study of patients on bisphosphonates, in conjunction with periodontal disease surgical treatment and, in some cases, implants, showed higher levels of attachment and greater BMD in the exposed group.[14]

In recent years, with the adverse effects of bisphosphonates in the craniomaxillofacial region widely reported, the general effects of these drugs on the region are being further investigated. The radiologic effects of bisphosphonates on the craniofacial skeleton have been explored.[15] The action of bisphosphonates on oral keratinocytes might give insight into how oral tissues might be compromised by the effects of bisphosphonates. Inhibition of oral mucosal cell healing has been investigated.[16] The possibility that a direct toxic effect of bisphosphonates on oral mucosa is playing a role on the oral effects of these medications is currently being investigated.[17]

An experimental animal model for bisphosphonate effect on alveolar bone is in development. Allen and Burr[18] report on the histologic observation of osteonecrosis in a placebo-controlled beagle dog study after 3 years of therapeutic level of exposure to alendronate. Their study demonstrates a selective effect of bisphosphonates on alveolar bone, showing increased density, loss of blood supply, and necrosis. An absolute decrease in the number of canaliculi is associated with lacunae empty of osteocytes. Ghost lacunae may also be a predictor of eventual clinical osteonecrosis.

OSTEONECROSIS OF THE JAWS

The first peer-reviewed publication by Ruggiero and collegeagues[19] in 2004 was a case series of

63 patients with osteonecrosis after exposure to intravenous or oral bisphosphonates, 87% of whom had received intravenous zoledronic acid or pamidronate. Subsequent to that report of a case series, other case series, as well as cohort studies and those with prospective design, have confirmed the reality of bisphosphonate-related osteonecrosis of the jaws (BRONJ). Although BRONJ is thought to represent osteonecrosis as a primary finding, osteomyelitis, soft tissue cellulitis, and periostitis with subperiosteal bone reaction occur concomitantly (**Fig. 2**).

The association between intravenous bisphosphonate use and BRONJ is well established, with incidence of between 1% and 10% of patients receiving these medications for an average of approximately 14 months. The information with regard to oral bisphosphonates and BRONJ risk is less clear. Some studies have demonstrated only cases from intravenous bisphosphonates or as few as 3% to 5% from oral bisphosphonates.[20] In an assessment of 840 patients on oral bisphosphonates, no cases of BRONJ were identified.[21] These drugs are replete in the older population that might have a jaw complication where bone necrosis and exposure, especially of tori and after extraction, have been known phenomenon long before bisphosphonates were prescribed. By 2005, Schwabe and Ziegler reported there were 129 million doses of oral bisphosphonates prescribed annually.[22] The ubiquitous nature of these drugs requires that comparative groups of patients exposed to bisphosphonates and a cohort population are examined. A mail survey in Australia of oral bisphosphonate patients revealed a possible rate of BRONJ of approximately 1 in 2200 patients with an average use of just over 2 years before presenting with symptoms.[23] In a survey of American Association of Oral and Maxillofacial Surgeons members reported in the *Journal of Oral and Maxillofacial Surgery*, 1700 surgeons reported 4700 cases of BRONJ.[24] The prevalence of BRONJ in oral bisphosphonate patients is difficult to determine due to the decreased supervision of these patients compared with oncology patients and the lack of a complete drug database. Health insurance claims studies can, however, be done. For example, of 179,784 patients on oral bisphosphonates, 43 had a medical claim for jaw surgery for inflammatory or necrotic condition.[25] In an Kaiser Permanente Oakland Medical Center study, Predicting Risk of Osteonecrosis of the Jaw with Oral Bisphosphonate Exposure (PROBE), the PROBE Investigators attempt to assess prevalence of BRONJ but with only a study of 952 exposed patients at this point in the peer-reviewed literature.[26] Their recent work demonstrates a modest increased risk as well with more years of use. There are also comparative studies of similar postmenopausal osteoporosis patients. A trial of once-yearly zoledronic acid enrolled 7714 patients and reported 1 case of osteonecrosis of the jaw in the study group and 1 in the placebo group over 3 years.[27] A survey of German patients reported only 1 case in 100,000 patient years, not demonstrating an association between oral bisphosphonate use and BRONJ.[28] In an assessment up to 2006, there were fewer than 50 cases attributable to oral bisphosphonates.[29] Yet clinicians today continue to see these cases. In my Oregon Health and Science University practice, 6 of 8 current stage 3 BRONJ patients are those with only oral bisphosphonate exposure.

The specific drug used may or may not play a role, with more oral use cases associated with alendronate (but with the greatest market share).[30] Zoledronate has also been reported more frequently with BRONJ, but dosing has changed since the drug began use and current studies seem to indicate that cases of BRONJ are consistent with use compared with pamidronate. Although no cases of BRONJ were initially reported with non-nitrogen bisphosphonates, such as clodronate or with denosumab (an antiosteoclast drug with another mode of action), these too have now been reported but incidence is less clear.[31] A single case report of osteonecrosis with clodrondate was not a severe case.[32] With denosumab used for breast cancer, a similar or higher incidence of osteonecrosis occurred compared with zoledronic acid.[33]

Approximately 5 out of 6 patients with osteonecrosis represent patients with malignancy. Based on route of administration and potency of the agent, effective dosage of bisphosphonates might

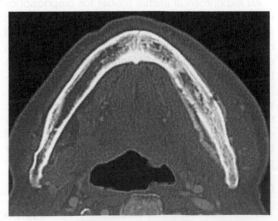

Fig. 2. Subperiosteal bone deposition in BRONJ.

be 4 to 12 times greater in metastatic cancer patients compared with osteoporosis patients.[34] In addition to the higher effective dose given over a shorter period, patients with malignancy suffer from a host of cofactors that also initiate or exacerbate their evolution of osteonecrosis. It is important to assess the cofactors of bisphosphonate use that make these patients at risk for BRONJ. Some of these are

1. The presence of tumor in bone
2. Anemia of malignancy affecting oxygen carrying capacity
3. Cachexia of malignancy effecting nutrition
4. Smoking and other pulmonary compromise
5. Chemotherapy
6. Radiation
7. Steroids
8. Increased metabolic load.

Cofactors also play a role in BRONJ in oral bisphosphonate patients.[35] Rheumatoid arthritis and associated antimetabolic medications, smoking, and diabetes play a role. Essentially any disease that adversely affects cellular metabolism, immune response, and oxygenation can be an important cofactor.

Obesity, long known as a factor in osteomyelitis of long bones and jaw, may be a factor in BRONJ as well.[36]

ORAL RISK FACTORS IN BRONJ

Strong evidence exists that tooth extraction is important in initiating BRONJ, although cause and effect are difficult to establish.[23,37] Approximately one-third to one-half of reported cases of BRONJ are associated with dental extraction.[38] Extraction, implants, and invasive periodontal therapy are the recognized procedural risk factors for the initiation of BRONJ.[39] A personal survey of more than 400 cases did not demonstrate any cases where direct dental restoration, indirect restoration, orthograde endodontic therapy, dental prophylaxis, or other preventive dental care has been associated with initiation of BRONJ. A rubber dam clamp has been associated, however, with developing BRONJ.[40] Case reports of nonsurgical and surgical root canal therapy initiating BRONJ have been reported.[41]

STAGING AND TREATING BRONJ

Understanding the sages of BRONJ can serve as a guide to treatment and assessing outcomes. The American Association of Oral and Maxillofacial Surgeons recently updated their assessment of BRONJ and now have 4 stages of the disease.[42]

Stage 0

There is no evidence of necrotic bone, but there are nonspecific clinical findings and symptoms. Although these findings can be in any stage of BRONJ, they are not associated with exposed bone in stage 0 patients. These findings may include

1. Odontalgia: in the absence of identifiable local cause due to caries, periodontal disease, hyperocclusion, and so forth
2. Bone pain: ischemic bone pain or that associated with inflammation at the site
3. Sinus pain: reactive sinusitis can be associated with inflammation or necrosis of bone
4. Paresthesia/dysesthesia: compressive neuropathy can be seen in the region of foramina, especially the inferior alveolar canal parts
5. Neuropathic pain: pain responsive to neurotropic agents, such as gabapentin, can be due to inflammatory or compressive nerve injury
6. Loosening of teeth: associated with diffuse bone loss not explained by usual periodontal causes
7. Periapical/periodontal fistula: presence of a fistula indicates necrotic bone from BRONJ or other common dental causes
8. Postextraction persistent dry socket: dry socket symptoms that persist more than 6 weeks.

Radiographic Findings in Stage 0

1. Alveolar bone loss
2. Bone resorption
3. Changes in trabecular pattern: dense woven bone and persistence of nonremodeled bone in extractions sockets
4. Thickening/obscuring of PDL: thickening of the lamina dura and decreased size of the periodontal ligament space
5. Inferior alveolar canal narrowing[43]
6. PET scans and other nuclear bone scans may be of value in assessing stage 0 patients and may be predictive of progression.[44]

Stage 1

There is exposure of bone with the absence of pain or evidence of infection (**Fig. 3**).

Stage 2

There is exposed and necrotic bone associated with infection as evidenced by pain and erythema in region of exposed bone with or without purulent drainage.

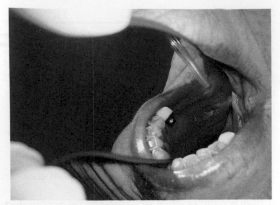

Fig. 3. Stage 1 BRONJ in the most frequent region, internal oblique ridge of the mandible.

Stage 3

There is exposed and necrotic bone in patients with pain, infection, and 1 or more of the following: exposed and necrotic bone extending beyond the region of alveolar bone (ie, inferior border and ramus in the mandible, maxillary sinus, and zygoma in the maxilla), resulting in pathologic fracture, extraoral fistula, oral antral/oral nasal communication, or osteolysis extending to the inferior border of the mandible or sinus floor.

Patients change stages during the course of BRONJ and can progress from stage 0 to stage 3 (**Fig. 4**).

Using the AAOMS guidelines can be helpful in assessing and making treatment decisions about patients with BRONJ. The most important feature of treatment planning is placing BRONJ in the context of a patient's overall illness and providing treatment that gives the greatest overall benefit. Many of the patients with the worst oral conditions are those least able to undergo extensive surgical care. Thus, the goals of treatment should be to provide mitigation of pain and loss of function while eliminating BRONJ when feasible. Advances in medical management can serve as adjuncts or exclusive treatments for BRONJ patients.

Withdrawal of bisphosphonate use, when in a patient's best interest, is helpful in affording improvement. Progress to stage 0 is especially likely in oral bisphosphonate patients for whom the drug is withdrawn.[45] The question of drug withdrawal must be considered in the context of the consequence of removal. Temporary withdrawal of bisphosphonate therapy for alendronate patients with osteoporosis does not have known adverse clinical effect but the long-term effects of permanent removal remain unknown.[46] If BRONJ is seen as equivalent to another SRE,

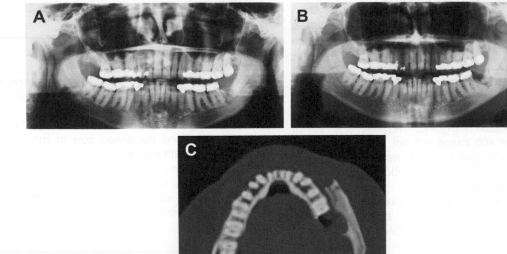

Fig. 4. (A) Progression of BRONJ over time in a patient with 2 years of Zometa use and metastatic breast cancer. Third molar was removed and dry socket packed in 2007. Treatment included medical management and sequestrectomies. (B) Note sequestration and sclerosis of left ramus (October 2009). (C) Pathologic fracture; note continued sclerosis on affected side and concurrent undisturbed asymptomatic side of mandible (2011).

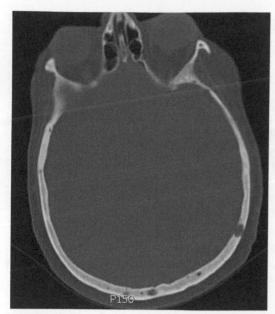

Fig. 5. Effects of breast cancer and 3 years of zoledronic acid treatment: loss of diploic layer, increased density, and focal metastases.

collagen in the urine (via C-terminal telopeptide), the effects of bisphosphonates in bone are long-standing. For example, see the changes in the skulls of 2 patients with BRONJ in **Figs. 5** and **6**.

The effect of withdrawal does depend on which bisphosphonate is used and for how long. It is thought that patients recover better from oral bisphosphonate use. One study of oral BRONJ related to the use of oral bisphosphonates, 11 of 30 patients resolved signs and symptoms spontaneously on withdrawal of alendronate.[45]

Management of stage 0 requires symptomatic treatment of existing signs and symptoms, consideration of a course of systemic antibiotic therapy, and consideration of withdrawal of bisphosphonate use if the benefits of that action outweigh the risks to the targeted disease.

Stage 1 disease patients are not suffering from associated infection due to the lack of redness, pus, swelling, or other systemic signs of infection. Topical use of 0.12% chlorhexidine is recommended to reduce the biofilm burden at the site of exposed bone and makes progression to stage 2 to 3 less likely. Direct application and friction removal of biofilm makes the use of toothbrush or gauze saturated with chlorhexidine a good method for many patients where additional mechanical damage can be avoided.

Stage 2 requires the addition of systemic antibiotics either orally or parenterally. Penicillin is the drug of choice in that it effectively addresses the oral organisms as well as BRONJ-specific organisms, such as *Actinomyces* and *Eikenella corrodens*. Although oral antibiotics can obtain sufficient blood levels for this purpose, compliance can waver and risk of various antibiotic-induced

such as fracture of hip or spine, then effectively treating BRONJ that causes another SRE is not effective treatment. Continued use of once-yearly zoledronate, for example, can protect against 40% to 70% of osteoporotic fracture, and for cancer patients, once-monthly administration reduces SREs 10% to 30%.[4] If patients are not at high risk of developing an SRE, however, temporary withdrawal of the drug is to be strongly considered. In spite of the ability to measure type I

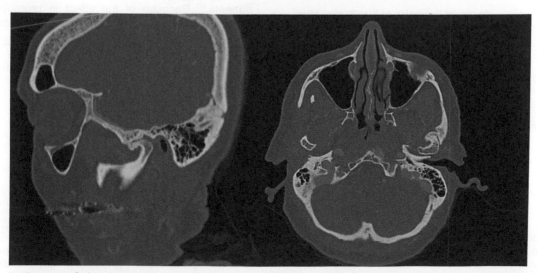

Fig. 6. Six years of alenronate with condylar changes and thickening of the skull.

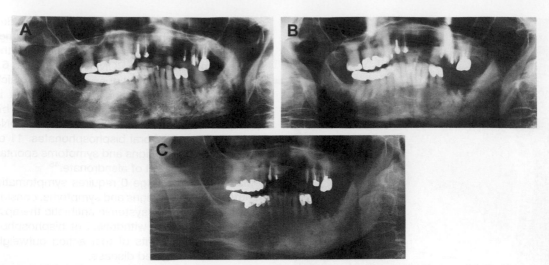

Fig. 7. (*A*) Patient with 3 years of alendronate, severe stage 3 BRONJ with pathologic fracture. (*B*) Five months of Forteo (June 2010). (*C*) One-year treatment with Forteo daily and systemic antibiotics, now stage 0.

gastrointestinal problems can ensue. In many cases, home intravenous use of antibiotics is needed for long duration. Antibiotic therapy should be continued as long as patients are in stage 2 and for a reasonable period after signs and symptoms have resolved. During the course of medical management of stage 2, sequestrectomy or other local débridement and extraction of teeth may be required. Extractions performed of patients with BRONJ should include careful surgical remodeling of bone (alveoplasty) and good adaptation of tissues because the ability of patients to remodel the extraction site is markedly inhibited.

Stage 3 is managed either medically or with surgical excision and reconstruction. In my practice, approximately 20% of patients progress to

stage 3 and require removal of a major affected part. Use of bone grafting methods that require osteoclasts for phase 2 bone healing seem unwise because remodeling of the graft is substantially inhibited.[47] The use of free tissue transfer is in wide use for this purpose and has reported good outcomes.[48]

Outcomes of medical therapy for BRONJ are promising, demonstrating equal outcomes comparing antibiotic therapy with surgical extirpation.[49]

The idea that surgery is a mainstay treatment for BRONJ ignores evidence that medical management, including innovative methods, is showing promising results.

Subcutaneous administration of parathormone is being investigated for use in noncancer BRONJ patients.[50] Because of the effect in promoting parathormone-producing tumors, it is not recommended for oncology patients. As a therapy in conjunction with other supportive therapy in compromised patients, I have found it effective.

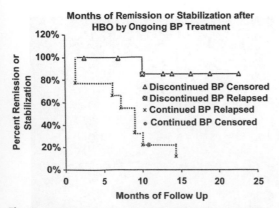

Months of Remission or Stabilization after HBO by Ongoing BP Treatment

△ Discontinued BP Censored
⊠ Discontinued BP Relapsed
✕ Continued BP Relapsed
○ Continued BP Censored

Percent Remission or Stabilization (y-axis)
Months of Follow Up (x-axis)

Fig. 8. Hyperbaric oxygen with and without continuing bisphosphonate treatment. (*From* Freiberger JJ, Padilla-Burgos R, Chhoeu AH, et al. Hyperbaric oxygen and bisphosphonate induced osteonecrosis of the jaw: a case series. J Oral Maxillofac Surg 2007;65(7); 1321–7; with permission.)

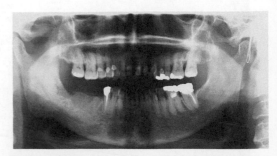

Fig. 9. Postextraction pain and thickening of periodontal ligament and hyperostosis right mandible with no exposed bone.

Name	Age	ONJ Stage	Treatment
Mary	87	3	Mand.Res.
Konni	54	3	Debride
William	87	3	Chlorhex
Mary	69	3	Max.res.
Diana	71	3	Forteo
Cora	72	3	Max.res.
June	82	3	Forteo
Dorothy	85	3	Debride

Fig. 10. My stage 3 oral bisphosphonate–related BRONJ patients, 3 of 8 resected (January 2011).

In an elderly patient with stage 3 BRONJ and pathologic fracture, treatment (substitution for alendronate) with Forteo (teriparatide) daily and supportive therapy with chlorhexidine and penicillin resulted in a stage 0 state at 1 year. This has the advantage of allowing the continued treatment of osteoporosis with Forteo, an approved drug for osteoporosis as well (**Fig. 7**).

Hyperbaric oxygen therapy and withdrawal of bisphosphonate with supportive care results in remission or stabilization of BRONJ affected sites as well as improvement of symptoms (**Fig. 8**).[51] The mechanism of hyperbaric oxygen is to improve ischemia at the site, promote angiogenesis, and address the anaerobic bacterial environment. Its use in metastatic cancer patients remains controversial.

Substituting non-nitrogen bisphosphonates for bisphosphonates has been considered as a therapy. By replacing alendronate with clodronate, displacement of the nitrogen component from bone might change the acidity of the local environment.[52] Parathormone is being evaluated as a factor in the pathogenesis and course of BRONJ.

Treatment of stage 0 patients will likely grow, as more such patients are identified and present with more readably identifiable imaging and clinical findings (**Fig. 9**). The future will offer more alternatives to treatment with bisphosphonates for patients with BRONJ as well as better nonsurgical management of BRONJ. This will be due to development of a greater understanding of the pathology of this vexing clinical problem. In my practice, even stage 3 patients in the winter of 2011 are for the most part managed medically (**Fig. 10**).

REFERENCES

1. Morgan G, Lipton A. Antitumor effects and anticancer actions of bisphosphonates [review]. Semin Oncol 2010;37(Suppl 2):S30–40.

2. Yamashita J, Koi K, Yang DY, et al. Effect of zoledronate on oral wound healing in rats. Clin Cancer Res 2011;17(6):1405–14.

3. Available at: http://www.nof.org/aboutosteoporosis/bonebasics/whybonehealthviewed. Accessed December 28, 2010.

4. Black DM, Delmas PD, Eastell R, et al. Once yearly Zolendronic Acid for treatment of postmenapausal osteoporosis. N Engl J Med 2007;356:1809–22.

5. Shane E. Evolving data about subtrochanteric fractures and bisphosphonates. N Engl J Med 2010;362(19):1825–7. Available at: http://www.answers.com/topic/bisphosphonate#ixzz1BJn7ZVc2. Accessed May 25, 2011.

6. Byrjalsen I, Leeming DJ, Qvist P, et al. Bone turnover and bone collagen maturation in osteoporosis: effects of antiresorptive therapies. Osteoporos Int 2008;19(3):339–48.

7. Fleisch H. Development of bisphosphonates. Breast Cancer Res 2002;4(1):30–4. Available at: http://www.answers.com/topic/bisphosphonate#ixzz1BJLqrvas. Accessed May 25, 2011.

8. FDA Approves Actonel (Risedronate) For Osteoporosis. Available at: http://www.pslgroup.com/dg/1cd17e.htm. Accessed May 25, 2011.

9. Roche our history. Available at: http://www.roche.com/home/company/com_hist/com_hist_2001.htm. Accessed May 25, 2011.

10. Adler RA. Osteoporosis in Men: what has changed? Curr Osteoporos Rep 2010;9(1):31–5.

11. Gnant M, Hadji P. Prevention of bone metastases and management of bone health in early breast cancer. Breast Cancer Res 2010;12(6):216.

12. Statement by Merck & Co., Inc. Regarding FOSAMAX® (alendronate sodium) and Rare Cases of Osteonecrosis of the Jaw 2006;21:349. Available at: http://www.merck.com/newsroom/press_releases/product/fosamax_statement.html. Accessed May 25, 2011.

13. Jeffcoat MK. Safety of Oral Bisphosphonates, controlled studies of alveolar bone. Int J Oral Maxillofac Implants 2006;21(3):349–53.

14. Lane N, Armitage GC, Loomer P, et al. Bisphosphonate therapy improves the outcome of conventional periodontal treatment: results of a 12-month, randomized, placebo-controlled study. J Periodontol 2005; 76(7):1113–22.

15. Phal PM, Myall RW, Assael LA, et al. Imaging findings of bisphosphonate-associated osteonecrosis of the jaws. AJNR Am J Neuroradiol 2007;28(6):1139–45.

16. Landesberg R, Cozin M, Cremers S, et al. Inhibition of oral mucosal cell healing by bisphosphonates. J Oral Maxillofac Surg 2008;66(5):839–47.

17. Reid IR, Bolland MJ, Grey AB. Is bisphosphonate-associated osteonecrosis of the jaw caused by soft tissue toxicity? Bone 2007;41(3):318–20.

18. Allen MR, Burr DB. Mandible matrix necrosis in beagle dogs after 3 years of daily oral bisphosphonate treatment. J Oral Maxillofac Surg 2008;66(5):987–94.

19. Ruggiero SL, Mehrotra B, Rosenberg TJ, et al. Osteonecrosis of the jaws associated with the use of bisphosphonates: a review of 63 cases. J Oral Maxillofac Surg 2004;62:527–34.

20. Abu-Id MH, Warnke PH, Gottschalk J, et al. "Bisphossy jaws"—high and low risk factors for bisphosphonate induced osteonecrosis of the jaw. J Craniomaxillofac Surg 2008;36(2):95–103.

21. Murad OM, Arora S, Farag AF, et al. Bisphosphonates and osteonecrosis of the jaw: a retrospective study. Endocr Pract 2007;13:232–8.

22. Schwabe U, Ziegler R. Mineralstoffpräparate und Osteoporosemittel. In: Schwabe U, Paffrath D, editors. Arzneiverordnungsreport 2005. Berlin (Heidelberg): Springer; 2005:755e756.

23. Mavrokokki T, Cheng A, Stein B, et al. Nature and frequency of bisphosphonate-associated osteonecrosis of the jaws in Australia. J Oral Maxillofac Surg 2007;65:415–23.

24. Ruggiero SL, Dodson TB, Assael LA, et al. American Association of Oral and Maxillofacial Surgeons Position Paper on Bisphosphonate-Related Osteonecrosis of the Jaws –2009 Update. J Oral Maxillofac Surg 2005;67(5 Suppl 1):2–12.

25. Cartsos VM, Zhu S, Zavras AI, et al. Bisphosphonate use and the risk of adverse jaw outcomes a medical claims study of 714,217 people. J Am Dent Assoc 2008;139(1):23–30.

26. Lo JC, O'Ryan FS, Gordon NP, et al, Predicting Risk of Osteonecrosis of the Jaw with Oral Bisphosphonate Exposure (PROBE) Investigators. Prevalence of osteonecrosis in Patients with Oral Bisphosphonate Exposure. J Oral Maxillofac Surg 2010;68(2): 243–53.

27. Grbic JT, Landesberg R, Lin SQ, et al, Health Outcomes Reduced Incidence With Zoledronic Ácid Once Yearly Pivotal Fracture Trial Research Group. Incidence of osteonecrosis of the jaw in women with postmenopausal osteoporosis in the health outcomes and reduced incidence with zoledronic acid once yearly pivotal fracture trial. J Am Dent Assoc 2008;139(1):32–40.

28. Felsenberg D, Hoffmeister B, Amling M. [Onkologie: Kiefernekrosen nach hoch dosierter Bisphosphonattherapie]. Peter Dtsch Arztebl 2006;103(46):A-3078 / B-2681 / C-2572 [in German].

29. Woo SB, Hellstein JW, Kalmar JR. Bisphosphonates and osteonecrosis of the jaws. Ann Intern Med 2006; 144:753–6 [erratum: Ann Intern Med 2006;145:235].

30. Van den Wyngaert T, Huizing MT, Vermorken JB. Bisphosphonates and osteonecrosis of the jaw: cause and effect or a post hoc fallacy? Ann Oncol 2006;17: 1197–204.

31. Diel IJ, Fogelman I, Al-Nawas B, et al. Pathophysiology, risk factors and management of bisphosphonate-associated osteonecrosis of the jaw: is there a diverse relationship of amino- and nonaminobisphosphonates? Crit Rev Oncol Hematol 2007;64(3):198–207.

32. Crépin S, Laroche ML, Sarry B, et al. Osteonecrosis of the Jaw induced by clodronate: a case report [Review]. Eur J Clin Pharmacol 2010;66(6):547–54.

33. Stopeck AT, Lipton A, Body JJ, et al. Denosumab compared with zoledronic acid for the treatment of bone metastases in patients with advanced breast cancer: a randomized, double-blind study. J Clin Oncol 2010;28(35):5132–9.

34. Bilezikian JP. Osteonecrosis of the jaw—do bisphosphonates pose a risk? N Engl J Med 2006; 355(22):2278–81. Available at: www.nejm.org. Accessed November 30, 2006.

35. Khosla S, Burr D, Cauley J, et al. Bisphosphonate associated osteonecrosis of the jaw: report of a taskforce for the American Society of bone and Mineral Research. J Bone Miner Res 2007;22(10):1479–91.

36. Wessel J, Dodson T, Zafras A. Zoledronate, smoking, and obesity are strong risk factors for osteonecrosis of the jaw: a case-control study. J Oral Maxillofac Surg 2008;66:625.

37. Yarom N, Yahalom R, Shoshani Y, et al. Osteonecrosis of the jaw induced by orally administered bisphosphonates: incidence, clinical features, predisposing factors and treatment outcome. Osteoporos Int 2007;18(10):1363–70.

38. Hoff AO, Toth BB, Altundag K, et al. The frequency and risk factors associated with osteonecrosis of the jaw in cancer patients treated with intravenous bisphosphonates. J Bone Miner Res 2008;6:826.

39. Gutta R, Louis PJ. Bisphosphonates and osteonecrosis of the jaws: science and rationale. Oral Surg Oral Med Oral Pathol Oral Radiol Endod 2007; 104(2):186–93.

40. Gallego L, Junquera L, Pelaz A, et al. Rubber dam clamp trauma during endodontic treatment: a risk factor of bisphosphonate-related osteonecrosis of the jaw? J Oral Maxillofac Surg 2011;69(6): e93–5.

41. Fugazzotto PA, Lightfoot S. Bisphosphonate osteonecrosis of the jaws and endodontic treatment. J Mass Dent Soc 2006;55(2):5.

42. Ruggiero SL, Dodson TB, Assael LA, et al. American Association of Oral and Maxillofacial Surgeons position paper on bisphosphonate-related osteonecrosis of the jaws—2009 update. J Oral Maxillofac Surg 2009;67(Suppl 1):2–12.

43. Arce K, Assael LA, Weissman JL. Imaging findings in bisphosphonate related osteonecrosis of the jaws. J Oral Maxillofac Surg 2009;67(Suppl 5):75–84.

44. Catalano L, Del Vecchio S, Petruzziello F, et al. Sestamibi and FDG-PET scans to support diagnosis of jaw osteonecrosis. Ann Hematol 2007;86(6):415–23.

45. Marx RE, Cillo JE Jr, Ulloa JJ. Oral bisphosphonate-induced osteonecrosis: risk factors, prediction of risk using serum CTX testing, prevention, and treatment. J Oral Maxillofac Surg 2007;65(12):2397–410.

46. Black DM, Schwartz AV, Ensrud KE, et al. Effects of continuing or stopping alendronate after 5 years of treatment the Fracture Intervention Trial Long-term Extension (FLEX): a randomized trial. JAMA 2006; 296:2927–38.

47. Assael L. Oral bisphosphonates as a cause of bisphosphonate-related osteonecrosis of the jaws: clinical findings, assessment of risks, and preventive strategies. J Oral Maxillofac Surg 2009;67(Suppl 5): 35–43.

48. Seth R, Futran ND, Alam DS, et al. Outcomes of vascularized bone graft reconstruction of the mandible in bisphosphonate-related osteonecrosis of the jaws. Laryngoscope 2010;120(11):2165–71.

49. Montebugnoli L, Felicetti L, Gissi DB, et al. Biphosphonate-associated osteonecrosis can be controlled by nonsurgical management. Oral Surg Oral Med Oral Pathol Oral Radiol Endod 2007; 104(4):473–7.

50. Harper RP, Fung E. Resolution of bisphosphonate-associated osteonecrosis of the mandible: possible application for intermittent low-dose parathyroid hormone [rhPTH(1-34)]. J Oral Maxillofac Surg 2007;65(3):573–80.

51. Freiberger JJ, Padilla-Burgos R, Chhoeu AH, et al. Hyperbaric Oxygen and bisphosphonate induced osteonecrosis of the jaw: a case series. J Oral Maxillofac Surg 2007;65(7):1321–7.

52. Yamaguchi K, Oizumi T, Funayama H, et al. Osteonecrosis of the jawbones in 2 osteoporosis patients treated with nitrogen-containing bisphosphonates: osteonecrosis reduction replacing NBP with non-NBP (etidronate) and rationale. J Oral Maxillofac Surg 2010; 68(4):889–97.

Osteoradionecrosis

Karla O'Dell, MD, Uttam Sinha, MD*

KEYWORDS

- Osteoradionecrosis • Head and neck cancer
- Fibroatrophy • Mandible

Osteoradionecrosis (ORN) of the mandible is a dire complication of radiation therapy for head and neck cancer. Radiation-induced osteonecrosis ranges from small asymptomatic bone exposures that remain stable for months to years and heals with conservative management, to severe necrosis with pathologic fracture necessitating surgical intervention and reconstruction. Symptoms can include pain, bad breath, dysgeusia, dysesthesia or anesthesia, trismus, difficulty with mastication, deglutition, and/or speech, fistula formation, pathologic fracture, and local, spreading, or systemic infection.[1]

ORN is defined as a condition in which irradiated bone becomes exposed through a wound in the overlying skin or mucosa and persists without healing for 3 to 6 months.[2,3] The exposed bone must occur in the absence of tumor recurrence, tumor necrosis during radiation therapy, or metastatic disease.[2] The incidence of ORN in the mandible following radiation treatment ranges from 2.6% to 15%.[1,4–9] The mean time from completion of radiation therapy to the development of ORN as reported in the literature ranges from 22 to 47 months.[9–13] This article reviews the anatomy, past and current theories of the pathophysiology, risk factors, and guidelines for prevention and treatment of postradiation ORN.

ANATOMY

The mandible is affected by ORN far more frequently than the other bones in the head and neck, although ORN of the maxilla, hyoid, and temporal bone have also been reported.[13] The mandible receives its blood supply from the inferior alveolar and facial arteries, and this external blood supply is markedly less than that in other facial bones.[14] In the mandible, the buccal cortex in the premolar, molar, and retromolar regions have been described as the most vulnerable sites for ORN. This vulnerability may be related to the posterior mandible consisting of denser bone with a higher mineral content and thus a higher absorbed radiation dose.[15] The mandible is also more likely to be in the field of radiation for treatment of oropharyngeal cancers. Grossly exposed necrotic bone is often seen in ORN. Histopathologic features of ORN are a mosaic of osteogenesis areas within extended areas of osteolysis.[7]

PATHOPHYSIOLOGY

The pathophysiology of ORN has been a controversial and evolving topic since it was first described in 1922 by Regaude.[16] Early experimental models of ORN showed evidence of bacteria in the tissue affected by ORN. Microscopic changes included loss of osteocytes and osteoblasts, and the filling of bony cavities with inflammatory cells (Fig. 1).[17] Interest in the role of bacteria in ORN gained popularity when in 1970 Meyer[18] defined the classic triad in the pathophysiology of ORN as radiation, trauma, and infection. He proposed that trauma, such as tooth removal, provided access for oral bacteria to enter the underlying bone, and the infection could then rapidly progress because the radiated bone had lost its resistance to bacterial infection. This process then resulted in radiation osteomyelitis.[18] Meyer's theory became the foundation for the use of antibiotics with surgery to treat ORN.

In 1983 Marx[3] challenged Meyer's theory, based on the observation that ORN did not have the clinical signs of infection, nor did it progress to sepsis in the same way osteomyelitis can, and occurred

Department of Otolaryngology- Head and Neck Surgery, University of Southern California, 1200 North State Street, Los Angeles, CA 90033, USA
* Corresponding author.
E-mail address: Sinha@usc.edu

Oral Maxillofacial Surg Clin N Am 23 (2011) 455–464
doi:10.1016/j.coms.2011.04.011
1042-3699/11/$ – see front matter © 2011 Published by Elsevier Inc.

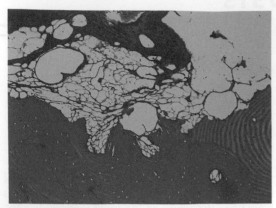

Fig. 1. Acellular bone in osteoradionecrosis, with loss of osteoblasts and osteoclasts.

in cases without trauma. He studied 26 cases of ORN and noted bacteria to only be on the surface of the bone and not in the necrotic area, indicating that microorganisms played a very minor role in the pathophysiology. Marx also noted that 35% of his cases could not be correlated with an episode of trauma. The histologic findings noted by Marx showed fibrosis of the mucosa, skin, and marrow space; hyalinization and thrombosis of vessels with loss of osteocytes and osteoblasts; and decreased vascularity of the connective tissue. The result is tissue that is hypovascular, hypocellular, and hypoxic compared with nonirradiated tissue.[3] Marx concluded that ORN is a problem of wound healing and is a disease process in both the bone and the enveloping soft tissue. He proposed the hypoxic-hypocellular-hypovascular theory, describing a 4-part sequence of: (1) radiation; (2) formation of hypoxic-hypovascular-hypocellular tissue; (3) tissue breakdown whereby collagen lysis and cellular death exceeds synthesis and cellular replication; and (4) chronic nonhealing wounds in which energy, oxygen, and structural precursor demand exceeds supply.[3] The major driving force in the pathogenesis was hypoxia, and these explanations formed the cornerstone for the use of hyperbaric oxygen in the treatment of ORN.

Recent advances in cellular and microbiology have allowed for the development of a new theory in the pathogenesis of ORN, the radiation-induced fibroatrophic theory.[19] The radiation-induced fibroatrophic theory suggests that the key event in the progression of ORN is the activation and deregulation of fibroblastic activity that leads to atrophic tissue within a previously radiated area. The hypothesis focuses on defective radiated bone and the imbalance between tissue synthesis and degradation in 3 distinct phases: (1) the prefibrotic phase, (2) the continuative organized phase, and

(3) the late fibroatrophic phase.[20] In the initial prefibrotic phase, radiation-induced injury to endothelial cells occurs together with the acute inflammatory response. The endothelial cell injury occurs from the direct damage by radiation and from the indirect damage by radiation-generated production of free radicals. Endothelial cell injury results in the release of cytokines that trigger an acute inflammatory response and result in a further release of reactive oxygen species (ROS). In the continuative organized phase the ROS release cytokines such as tumor necrosis factor α (TNF-α), platelet-derived growth factor, fibroblast growth factor β, interleukin (IL)-1, IL-4, and IL-6, and transforming growth factor β1, resulting in abnormal fibroblastic activity causing disorganization of the extracellular matrix. During the late fibroatrophic healing phase, an attempted tissue remodeling occurs with the formation of fragile healed tissues that are vulnerable to reactivated inflammation in the event of local injury.[21] The end result is hypocellular bone and reduced bone matrix formation compensated by fibrosis.[7] Based on this theory, new treatment regimens targeting ROS and radiation-induced fibrosis have been developed.[20]

CLASSIFICATION

There have been several classification systems suggested to determine the severity of ORN to guide treatment.[1,2,22] Marx's initial classification system was widely used but was limited because it was based on clinical response to a specific treatment, namely hyperbaric oxygen therapy (HBOT).[22] Other staging systems reflected the progress of the disease (ie, Stage I—resolving, Stage II—chronic persistent, Stage III—progressive).[1] Schwartz and Kagan[2] proposed a staging system based on clinical assessment and physical findings (**Table 1**). Clinical Stage I is superficial involvement of the bone in which only the exposed cortical bone is necrotic and soft tissue ulceration is minimal (**Fig. 2**). The majority of Stage I ORN resolves with conservative management. Stage II is localized involvement of the exposed cortical bone, with the underlying portions of the medullary bone also being necrotic. It is divided into Stage IIa, with minimal soft tissue ulceration, and Stage IIb, with soft tissue necrosis, including orocutaneous fistula. The majority of Stage II ORN resolves with conservative management or minor surgical procedures. Stage III is diffuse involvement of the bone with full-thickness involvement, including the lower border of the mandible (**Fig. 3**). Pathologic fracture may occur, and all Stage III ORN patients require surgical intervention. Stage III is also subdivided, with Stage IIIa having minimal soft tissue ulceration

Table 1
Clinical staging of osteoradionecrosis

Stage	Description	Treatment
I	Superficial involvement, only cortical bone exposed Minimal soft tissue ulceration	Majority improve with conservative management
II a: Minimal soft tissue ulceration b: Soft-tissue necrosis	Localized involvement of mandible, exposed cortical and medullary bone are necrotic Possible orocutaneous fistula	Majority improve with conservative management, surgical procedures, or hyperbaric oxygen therapy
III a: Minimal soft tissue ulceration b: Soft tissue necrosis	Diffuse involvement of the mandible, including the lower border. Pathologic fracture may occur Possible orocutaneous fistula	Require surgical intervention, resection, and reconstruction

From Schwartz HC, Kagan AR. Osteoradionecrosis of the mandible: scientific basis for clinical staging. Am J Clin Oncol 2002;25(2):168–9; with permission.

and Stage IIIb having soft tissue necrosis, including orocutaneous fistula.

DIAGNOSIS

Diagnosis of ORN is based on symptoms and clinical examination. Clinical symptoms include pain, bad breath, trismus, and difficulties in chewing, swallowing, and speech. Areas of ulceration or necrosis of the skin or mucosa is also seen with exposed necrotic bone (see **Fig. 3**). The affected site is within the radiation treatment area.[1] Dental extractions, surgery, or other types of trauma frequently precede the onset of ORN[10]; however, the rate of spontaneous ORN with no precipitating trauma is 10% to 48% in the literature.[1,3,22–24] ORN is a result of impaired wound healing and not an infection like osteomyelitis, but the bone may become secondarily infected. Patients can present with orocutaneous fistulas (see **Fig. 3**) or pathologic fractures, but these do not have to be present for a diagnosis of ORN.[2,25] The possibility of recurrence of cancer must be excluded by performing an incisional biopsy.

Radiology

Imaging studies aid in diagnosis and help to distinguish ORN from tumor recurrence. Plain film panorex, computed tomography (CT) scan, magnetic resonance imaging (MRI), and bone scans are usually used for diagnosis of ORN. On panoramic radiography, mandibular ORN usually appears as inhomogeneous lytic areas, interspersed with zones of increased radiodensity (**Fig. 4**). It is sometimes associated with a pathologic fracture, and radiopaque sequestra may be seen.[26] A CT scan is more sensitive than panoramic radiography in detecting ORN and has the ability to show soft

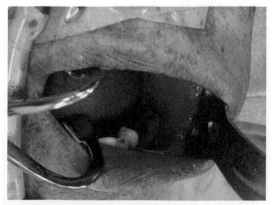

Fig. 2. Intraoral osteoradionecrosis with ulceration of mucosa and exposure of necrotic bone.

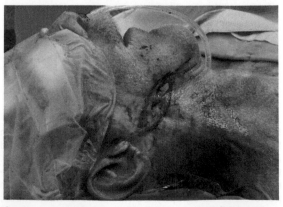

Fig. 3. Osteoradionecorosis with skin involvement.

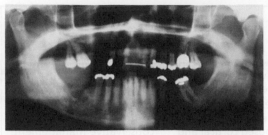

Fig. 4. Panoramic radiograph of 52-year-old patient with osteoradionecrosis after external beam radiation, showing defect in right body of the mandible.

tissue, which can help distinguish between bone destruction related to ORN and that associated with tumor recurrence.[27] Also on CT scans, interruptions in the cortical margins of the mandible are nearly always seen, and bone fragmentation is often present (**Fig. 5**). A few small pieces of bone appear separated from the remainder of the mandible.[28] MRI shows altered bone marrow signal intensities in the mandibular parts involved by ORN. These areas show abnormal, homogeneous, low-marrow signal intensity on T1-weighted images; increased signal intensity on T2-weighted images may also be observed.[26] On both MRI and CT scanning, the occurrence of abnormal findings distant or contralateral to the site of the primary tumor, and a long interval (>2 years) between primary tumor treatment and onset of symptoms suggest the diagnosis of ORN.[26]

Radionuclide bone scanning with technetium methylene diphosphonate can identify osteoblastic activity, and can detect bony changes earlier than conventional radiography.[13] It is useful in the diagnosis of ORN, but the scan remains

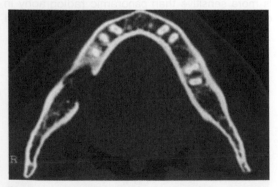

Fig. 5. Computed tomography scan of the patient in **Fig. 4**, showing thinning of the buccal cortex and a lingual defect in the right body of the mandible. (*From* Store G, Larheim TA. Mandibular osteoradionecrosis: a comparison of computed tomography with panoramic radiography. Dentomaxillofac Radiol 1999; 28:295–300; with permission.)

abnormal despite clinical improvement, and therefore has little utility in monitoring the clinical course. Gallium scans localize in the bone and inflammatory lesions. Gallium uptake has been shown to be of little use in the diagnosis of ORN, but does correlate with clinical findings following treatment. Persisting positive gallium scans may indicate the need for further treatment or surgery.[13]

RISK FACTORS

The development of ORN is dependent on many factors. These risk factors are associated with characteristics of the primary cancer, the treatment, and patient hygiene and habits (**Table 2**).

The site of the primary tumor influences the amount and location of mandible exposed to radiation, and has been shown to be associated with ORN development. ORN is most prevalent following radiation therapy for primary tumors of the oral tongue, floor of mouth, alveolar ridge, retromolar trigone, and tonsil.[5,9,10,12,23] This aspect relates to the large volume of mandible included in the primary radiation field in high-dose range for these tumor types, and the surgical approach to resection tumors in these sites often requires mandibular osteotomies or mandibulectomies that are traumatic to the bone tissue.[23] The risk of ORN is greater in patients with tumors of advanced stage.[5,9,10,23] Oh and colleagues[10]

Table 2 Risk factors associated with osteoradionecrosis	
Risk Factors	**Increased Risk of Osteoradionecrosis**
Location of primary tumor	Tongue, floor of mouth, alveolar ridge, retromolar trigone, tonsil
Stage of cancer	Stage III/IV
Dose of radiation	Doses >60 Gy
Prior surgery for primary tumor	Mandibulectomies or osteotomies before radiation
Oral hygiene	Periodontal disease; oral hygiene also influences response to treatment
Dental extractions	Extraction after radiation exposure
Alcohol use	Continued use during and after radiation therapy
Tobacco use	Continued use during and after radiation therapy
Nutritional status	Poor nutrition affects wound healing

reported that the number of ORN patients with advanced-stage tumors (Stage III or IV or recurrent disease) was 4.7 times greater than those with early-stage tumors (Stage I or II).

Initial treatment of the cancer related to surgical resection, dose of radiation, and concurrent chemotherapy influence the development of ORN. Surgical procedures to gain access to the tumor during surgery, including marginal mandibulectomy or mandibulotomy, increase the risk for ORN.[9] The risk of ORN is noted at radiation doses greater than 60 Gy.[9,12,29] In a retrospective study of 104 patients, Curi and Luciano[23] showed that few patients with radiation doses less than 50 Gy developed ORN, and the size of the ORN in the mandible was associated with increasing radiation doses.

Dental disease and dental extractions following radiation therapy are well-established predisposing factors to ORN.[4,5] Poor oral hygiene and dentition increase the likelihood of dental caries during radiation. Oral hygiene can also affect the healing of patients who develop ORN. Oh and colleagues[10] showed that patients with poor oral hygiene had a 3.06-times greater odds of ORN not resolving than patients with good oral hygiene. The nutritional status of the patient can also influence the progression of ORN.[30] Smoking and alcohol use during and after radiation therapy are risk factors for developing ORN.[4,5,23] Kluth and colleagues[4] retrospectively evaluated patients receiving definitive radiotherapy for head and neck malignancy, and compared the characteristics of those who developed ORN with those of patients who did not. It was confirmed that there was a significantly higher incidence of ORN associated with those who used alcohol or smoked during and/or after radiation. These habits increase the risk of mucosal breakdown, leading to ORN. Heavy tobacco and alcohol use is also associated with poor oral hygiene, which has also been shown to predispose patients to ORN.[4,5]

PREVENTION
Dental Care

Prevention of ORN involves minimizing the risk factors, including dental care and use of intensity-modulated radiation therapy (IMRT). Guidelines have been established for dental care before, during, and after radiation to minimize ORN.[31] Criteria for the extraction of teeth before radiation therapy include moderate to advanced periodontal disease (pocket-depth of more than 5 mm); extensive periapical lesions of the roots; extensive tooth decay; partially impacted or incompletely erupted teeth; and residual root tips not fully covered by bone or showing radiolucency.[31,32]

Deeply impacted teeth that are completely covered by bone and mucosa can be left without increased risk of late problems.[31] Dental extractions, removal of residual root tips, and removal of impacted teeth should be performed atraumatically with careful tissue handling, with alveolotomy and primary wound closure when possible. An interval of 2 to 3 weeks' healing time between tooth extraction and the onset of radiation therapy is recommended.[33] Dental screening before radiation therapy is aimed at preventing extractions of teeth from segments of the mandible already exposed to radiation.[34] It has been shown that dental extractions during or following radiation have a higher risk of developing ORN.[5,33] Maintaining good oral hygiene is very important before, during, and after radiation therapy. It is advised to have patients brush with high-fluoride toothpaste.[35] In addition to dental hygiene, use of topical fluoride applied in custom trays is indicated for patients with radiation-induced xerostomia.[30]

Role of Intensity-Modulated Radiation Therapy

IMRT allows for higher doses of radiation to be targeted at the tumor and minimizes collateral damage to the adjacent normal tissue.[36] Decreasing radiation exposure to the mandible has the potential to decrease ORN. Ahmed and colleagues[36] showed that IMRT decreased the total maximum radiation dose to the mandible and also decreased the volume of the mandible that was exposed to higher doses of 50, 55, and 60 Gy. In addition, decreased exposure to the parotid resulted in improved salivary gland flow and, therefore, decreased xerostomia and the potential for cavities as well as the need for dental extractions. This dosimetric advantage seen with IMRT can translate clinically into a lower incidence of ORN with IMRT therapy.

TREATMENT

Both medical and surgical management are used for ORN, depending on the severity of the condition. Medical management techniques include conservative management, including oral care, and local debridement, alone or combined with ultrasonography or hyperbaric oxygen. Surgical management involves resection of the necrotic bone and soft tissue with various reconstructions.

Conservative Management

Conservative management consists of avoidance of irritants such as tobacco, alcohol, and ill-fitting dentures as well as weekly physician visits that involve local debridement with antiseptic solutions including chlorhexidine, sodium iodide, and peroxide. Systemic antibiotics are saved for episodes of acute infection.[23] Fixation plates and screws are removed if they appear to be a contributing factor. Analgesics and anti-inflammatories are prescribed when necessary.[23] Simple management involves gentle removal of sequestra in lesions (a sequestrum is a piece of dead bone that has become separated from normal bone during the process of necrosis).[37] In one study simple management with removal of sequestra resulted in 75% of patients obtaining complete mucosal coverage, resulting in stable lesions.[25] Overall, conservative management leads to complete resolution of ORN in 42% to 48% of patients.[23,25]

Part of conservative management for ORN is the reduction of local irritants such as alcohol or tobacco. A retrospective study of 114 patients over 16 years found that patients who continued smoking after ORN diagnosis had a 2.35 times greater risk of their ORN not resolving with conservative management, compared with patients who did not continue to smoke.[10]

Hyperbaric Oxygen

Since first being introduced for use in ORN by Hart and Mainous[33] in 1975, HBOT has become an increasingly popular treatment for ORN. Recently, however, there has been some controversy regarding its effectiveness. During HBOT, patients breathe 100% oxygen at increased pressures (2–3 atm). This action results in the increase of the tissue oxygen pressure, leading to augmented endothelial cell and fibroblast proliferation.[38] In the long term it stimulates collagen synthesis, matrix deposition, angiogenesis, and epithelialization which, in turn, promotes wound healing.[39] HBOT is used in the treatment of ORN in a variety of clinical situations. It is used as part of conservative management or combined with surgical treatment, or may be applied prophylactically when a procedure, such as tooth extraction, is performed. Marx[22] was one of the initial proponents of HBOT for treatment of ORN. In 1983 he introduced a treatment protocol combining HBOT with surgery in 3 stages. Based on the response to therapy more extensive surgery is performed: from simple sequestrectomy with primary closure to resection with reconstruction. The use of HBOT before and after the procedure is the key to this treatment modality.[22] In a randomized trial Marx and colleagues[40] showed that HBOT before and after dental extraction, in previously radiated patients, decreased the risk of ORN in comparison with penicillin alone. The current protocol for HBOT

includes 20 to 30 dives at 2.0 to 2.5 atmospheres for 90 to 120 minutes at each session, once a day for 5 days. If a dental extraction or surgical procedure is performed, the patient takes an additional 10 dives.[6]

Complications of HBOT include Eustachian tube dysfunction, middle ear barotrauma, seizure, and decompression sickness. The main contraindications are optic neuritis and pulmonary disease.[41] Although in the past there have been concerns regarding hyperbaric oxygen stimulating malignant growth, there has been little evidence to support this and it should not be a concern of the prescribing physician.[42]

The use of HBOT is supported by many retrospective series and literature reviews. Feldmeier and Hampson[8] reviewed 14 published studies and noted that after HBOT there was improvement in 310 out of 371 (83.6%) patients with ORN. In a 2004 systematic literature search from 1960 to 2004, Pasquier and colleagues[43] concluded that despite the small number of controlled trials, HBOT may be indicated in the treatment of mandibular ORN in combination with surgery and during dental extraction.

Despite studies and reviews that show efficacy of HBOT, it remains a topic of debate in the treatment of ORN. The study by Annane and colleagues[24] in 2004 that questioned the effectiveness of HBOT was a randomized, placebo-controlled, double-blind trial from the ORN96 study. The study failed to show any beneficial effect of HBOT in patients with ORN. The trial was stopped early based on the lack of evidence that HBOT was better than placebo.[24] However, there were several critiques of the study including the fact that the study excluded patients with more advanced ORN as well as those with extension of ORN to the inferior border of the mandible or with a pathologic fracture. In addition, one of the outcomes in the study was the need for surgical resection, although many studies, including the Marx protocol, used HBOT in coordination with surgery as combined therapy; therefore it was claimed that the need for surgery does not necessarily indicate a treatment failure.[44,45] Despite the criticism this study has eroded some of the enthusiasm regarding HBOT in the treatment of ORN. The debate of HBOT is ongoing, with proponents both for and against its use.[41,45]

Ultrasound

The use of ultrasound has also been proposed as a conservative treatment for ORN and an alternative to HBOT.[46] The use of ultrasound in ORN was started after it was successfully used in the healing of ischemic varicose ulcers and fracture nonunions. It has been shown that ultrasound increases angiogenesis and stimulates collagen and bone production.[47] Harris[47] proposed a protocol of 40 to 50 10-minute sessions until healing is complete. Ultrasound can also be used as prophylaxis prior to postradiation dental extractions.[46]

Pentoxifylline-Tocopherol-Clodronate Combination

A new adjunctive treatment in ORN is the pentoxifylline-tocopherol-clodronate combination (Pentoclo).[7] Based on the radiation-induced fibrosis theory of ORN pathogenesis, this combination therapy targets radiation-induced bone fibrosis and stimulates osteogenesis via the antioxidant pathway. Pentoxifylline is a methlyxanthine derivative that exerts an anti–TNF-α effect, vasodilates, and inhibits inflammatory reactions. Tocopherol (vitamin E) scavenges the ROS generated during oxidative stress. These two drugs work synergistically as potent antifibrotic agents.[20] Clodronate is a biphosphonate that inhibits osteoclastic bone destruction and osteolysis.[20] In a recent phase-2 clinical trial,[7] 54 patients with refractory ORN were given a regimen of Pentoclo. The patients were given daily combination of pentoxifylline 800 mg/d, vitamin E 1000 IU/d, and clodronate 1600 mg/d from Monday to Friday. All 54 patients experienced a complete recovery over a median period of 9 months.[7] Although these results need to be confirmed with a randomized trial, this combination is a new option in the medical treatment of ORN.

Surgery

Indications for surgery in ORN include Stage III disease, involvement of the inferior borders of the mandible, pathologic fracture, and failed conservative management.[11] Surgery involves resection of all involved necrotic bone and soft tissue, and primary reconstruction. The extent of planned bony resection is initially based on preoperative imaging studies. However, the ultimate extent of resection is based on intraoperative findings. Resection is continued until the presence of healthy bleeding bone at the margin is identified (**Figs. 6** and **7**).[11,48] The majority of the intraoral mucosa can be preserved. Tetracycline bone fluorescence has also been proposed as a guide to pinpoint the margins of resection in ORN.[49]

After resection, reconstruction options include osseous or osteocutaneous microvascular free tissue transfer from a variety of sites including the fibula, scapula, and iliac crest. Myocutaneous rotational flaps, including the pectoralis major, are

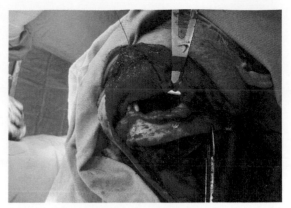

Fig. 6. Planned segmental mandibulectomy for osteoradionecrosis.

used rarely in patients who are poor surgical candidates.[50–52] First described for use in segmental mandible defects by Hidalgo[53] in 1988, the fibula osteocutaneous free flap is the most commonly used free flap for mandibular reconstruction in ORN. Based on the peroneal vessels, there are many features of the fibula that make it the best option for mandibular reconstruction. The fibula free flap has up to 25 cm of vascularized bone, which is an adequate length to reconstruct any segmental defect in the mandible. The periosteal blood supply is abundant and there is little variation in bone shape along the length of the graft, permitting multiple osteotomies to be performed as little as 1 cm apart, and allowing great flexibility in contouring the graft to simulate the shape of the mandible (**Fig. 8**).[53] Jacobson and colleagues[54] describe using a single fibular free flap for reconstruction of bilateral ORN of the mandible. The fibula has also proved to be a reliable flap, with 95% survival rate, and can be harvested using a 2-team approach, minimizing anesthesia time.[55] A decent aesthetic and functional reconstruction can be achieved using this

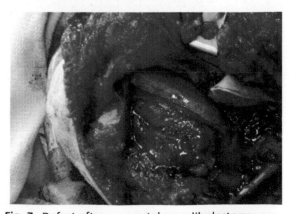

Fig. 7. Defect after segmental mandibulectomy.

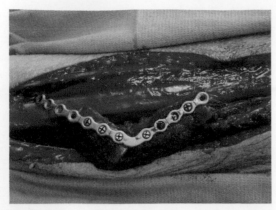

Fig. 8. Osseous fibula flap (bone only) harvested, contoured with osteotomies, and adapted to with mandible reconstruction bar before interrupting peroneal vessels.

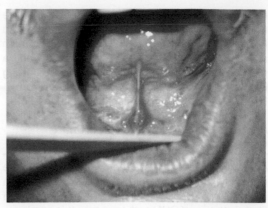

Fig. 10. Intraoral view of the same patient after segmental mandibulectomy with fibula free flap (bone only) reconstruction.

flap (**Figs. 9** and **10**). The iliac crest free flap has the benefit of height relative to the native mandible, which helps in oral competence but has increased morbidity at the donor site.[51] Because the extent of soft tissue defect is minimal during surgery for ORN, scapula free flap is rarely used for mandible reconstruction. Poor bone stock and the difficulty of positioning during harvest limit its use. This flap is used for those patients who have peripheral vascular disease and gait disturbance. Regardless of which donor site is used, the goals of mandible reconstruction are to reestablish the form of the lower third of the face and restore the patient's ability to eat, speak, and maintain a patent airway.

Several studies on free flap reconstruction of the mandible note a higher rate of complications in patients undergoing reconstruction for ORN.[11,48,52] Suh and colleagues[52] showed that there is an increased rate of complications in free

flaps for ORN with a possibility of recurrence after surgery.[11] This finding may be related to unspecific guidelines of how much bone is necessary for reconstruction.[52] Cannady and colleagues[56] noted an increased time interval between radiation and ORN development, and more extensive surgery up front resulted in higher flap failure and overall complications.

Despite the increased complication rate, resection with vascularized flap reconstruction may be the only option in advanced ORN. In addition, there is a 91% success rate in control of the ORN symptoms after free flap reconstruction of the mandible.[11] Patients with ORN report an overall improvement in quality of life after resection with free flap reconstruction, especially regarding decreased pain after surgery.[57,58]

SUMMARY

ORN can be a devastating complication of radiation therapy after treatment of head and neck cancer. While predisposing factors are clearly evident, there is an ongoing debate on how best to define and classify this disease process. There is also controversy regarding the best protocol for treatment, particularly the use of HBOT. New therapies focus on molecular biologic agents to prevent and treat ORN.

REFERENCES

1. Epstein JB, Wong FL, Stevenson-Moore P. Osteoradionecrosis: clinical experience and a proposal for classification. J Oral Maxillofac Surg 1987;45: 104–10.
2. Schwartz HC, Kagan AR. Osteoradionecrosis of the mandible: scientific basis for clinical staging. Am J Clin Oncol 2002;25(2):168–71.

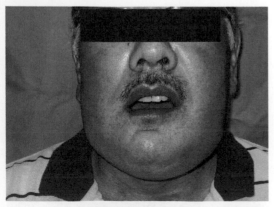

Fig. 9. Postoperative view after segmental mandibulectomy with fibula free flap.

3. Marx R. Osteoradionecrosis: a new concept in its pathophysiology. J Oral Maxillofac Surg 1983; 41:283–8.

4. Kluth E, Jain PR, Stuchell RN, et al. A study of factors contributing to the development of osteoradionecrosis of the jaws. J Prosthet Dent 1988;59(2): 194–201.

5. Reuther T, Schuster T, Mende U, et al. Osteoradionecrosis of the jaws as a side effect of radiotherapy of head and neck tumor patients- a report of a thirty year retrospective review. Int J Oral Maxillofac Surg 2003;32:289–95.

6. Dhanda J, Hall TJ, Wilkens A. Patterns of treatment of osteoradionecrosis with hyperbaric oxygen therapy in the United Kingdom. Br J Oral Maxillofac Surg 2009;47:210–3.

7. Delanian S, Chatel C, Porcher R. Complete restoration of refractory mandibular osteoradionecrosis by prolonged treatment with a Pentoxifylline-Tocopherol-Clodronate Combination (PENTOCLO): a phase II trial. Int J Radiat Oncol Biol Phys 2011; 80(3):832–9.

8. Feldmeier JJ, Hampson NB. A systemic review of the literature reporting the application of hyperbaric oxygen prevention and treatment of delayed radiation injuries: an evidence based approach. Undersea Hyperb Med 2002;29(1):4–30.

9. Lee IJ, Woong SK, Chang GL, et al. Risk factors and dose-effect relationship for mandibular osteoradionecrosis in oral and oropharyngeal cancer. Int J Radiat Oncol Biol Phys 2009;75(4):1084–91.

10. Oh HK, Chambers M, Martin J, et al. Osteoradionecrosis of the mandible: treatment outcomes and factors influences the progress of osteoradionecrosis. J Oral Maxillofac Surg 2009;67:1378–86.

11. Alam DS, Nuara M, Christian J. Analysis of outcomes of vascularized flap reconstruction in patients with advanced mandibular osteoradionecrosis. Otolaryngol Head Neck Surg 2009;141:196–201.

12. Store G, Boysen M. Mandibular osteoradionecrosis clinical behavior and diagnostic aspects. Clin Otolaryngol Allied Sci 2000;25(5):378–84.

13. Epstein J, Wong FL, Dickens A. Bone and gallium scans in post radiation osteoradionecrosis of the jaws. Head Neck 1992;14:288–92.

14. Chrcanovic BR, Reher P, Sousa AA, et al. Osteoradionecrosis of the jaws—a current overview—part 1. Oral Maxillofac Surg 2010;14:3–16.

15. Morrish RB, Chan E, Silverman S, et al. Osteoradionecrosis in patients irradiated for head and neck carcinoma. Cancer 1981;47:1980–3.

16. Regaude C. [Sur la necrose des os attente par un processus cancereux et traits par les radiations]. Compt Rend Soc Bio 1922;87:629. Quoted in Oral Surg 1951:4 [in French].

17. Gowgiel JM. Experimental radiosteonecrosis of the jaws. J Dent Res 1960;39:176–97.

18. Meyer I. Infectious diseases of the jaws. J Oral Surg 1970;28:17.

19. Delanian S, Lefaix JL. The radiation-induced fibroatrophic process: therapeutic perspective via the antioxidant pathway. Radiother Oncol 2004;73: 119–31.

20. Delanian S, Depondt J, Lefaix JL. Major healing of refractory mandible osteoradionecrosis after treatment combining pentoxifylline and tocopherol: a phase II trial. Head Neck 2005;27:114–23.

21. Lyons A, Ghazali N. Osteoradionecrosis of the jaws: current understanding of its pathophysiology and treatment. Br J Oral Maxillofac Surg 2008;46: 653–60.

22. Marx RE. A new concept in the treatment of osteoradionecrosis. J Oral Maxillofac Surg 1983;41:351–7.

23. Curi MM, Luciano LD. Osteoradionecrosis of the jaws: retrospective study of the background factors and treatment in 104 cases. J Oral Maxillofac Surg 1997;35:540–4.

24. Annane D, Depondt J, Aubert P, et al. Hyperbaric oxygen therapy for radionecrosis of the jaw: a randomized, placebo-controlled double blind trial from the ORN96 study group. J Clin Oncol 2004; 22:4893–900.

25. Wong JK, Wood RE, McLean M. Conservative management of osteoradionecrosis. Oral Surg Oral Med Oral Pathol Oral Radiol Endod 1997;84:16.

26. Hermans R. Imaging of the mandible. Neuroimaging Clin N Am 2003;13(3):597–604.

27. Store G, Larheim TA. Mandibular osteoradionecrosis: a comparison of computed tomography with panoramic radiography. Dentomaxillofac Radiol 1999; 28:295–300.

28. Hermans R, Fossiont E, Ioanmides C. CT findings in osteoradionecrosis of the mandible. Skeletal Radiol 1996;25:31–6.

29. Bedwinek JM, Shukovsky LJ, Fletcher GH, et al. Osteoradionecrosis in patients treated with definitive radiotherapy for squamous cell carcinomas of the oral cavity and naso- and oropharynx. Radiology 1976;119:665–7.

30. Jacobson A, Buchbinder D, Hu K, et al. Paradigm shifts in the management of osteoradionecrosis of the mandible. Oral Oncol 2010;46:795–801.

31. Jansma J, Vissink A, Spijkervet FK, et al. Protocol for the prevention and treatment of oral sequelae resulting from head and neck radiation therapy. Cancer 1992;70:2171–80.

32. Bruins HH, Koole R, Jolly DE, et al. Pretherapy dental decisions in patients with head and neck cancer. A proposed model for dental decision support. Oral Surg Oral Med Pathol Oral Radiol Endod 1998;86:256–67.

33. Hart GB, Mainous EG. The treatment of radiation necrosis with hyperbaric oxygen. Cancer 1976;37: 2580–5.

34. Friedman RB. Osteoradionecrosis: causes and prevention. NCI Monogr 1990;9:145–9.

35. Joshi VK. Dental treatment planning and management for the mouth cancer patient. Oral Oncol 2010; 6:475–9.

36. Ahmed M, Hansen VN, Harrington KJ, et al. Reducing the risk of xerostomia and mandibular osteoradionecrosis: the potential benefits of intensity modulated radiotherapy in advanced oral cavity carcinoma. Med Dosim 2009;34(3):217–24.

37. Merriam-Webster online medical dictionary. 2010. Available at: www.merriam-webster.com/medical/sequestra. Accessed November 30, 2010.

38. Tompach PC, Lew D, Stoll JL. Cell response to hyperbaric oxygen treatment. Int J Oral Maxillofac Surg 1997;26:82–6.

39. Marx RE, Ehler WJ, Tayapongsak P, et al. Relationship of oxygen dose to angiogenesis induction in irradiated tissue. Am J Surg 1990;160:519–24.

40. Marx RE, Johnson RP, Kline SN. Prevention of osteoradionecrosis. A randomized prospective clinical trial of hyperbaric oxygen versus penicillin. J Am Dent Assoc 1985;111:49.

41. Bessereau J, Annane D. Treatment of osteoradionecrosis of the jaw: the case against the use of hyperbaric oxygen. J Oral Maxillofac Surg 2010; 68:1907–10.

42. Feldmeier JJ. Hyperbaric oxygen for delayed radiation injuries. Undersea Hyperb Med 2004;31:133–5.

43. Pasquier D, Hoelscher T, Schmutz J, et al. Hyperbaric oxygen therapy in the treatment of radioinduced lesions in normal tissues: a literature review. Radiother Oncol 2004;72:1–13.

44. Shaw RJ, Dhanda J. Hyperbaric oxygen in the management of late radiation injury to the head and neck. Part 1: treatment. Br J Oral Maxillofac Surg 2010. DOI:10.1016/j.bjoms.2009.10.036.

45. Freiberg JJ, Feldmeier JJ. Evidence supporting the use of hyperbaric oxygen in the treatment of osteoradionecrosis of the jaws. J Oral Maxillofac Surg 2010;68:1903–6.

46. Reher P, Harris M. Ultrasound for the treatment of osteoradionecrosis—letter to the editor. J Oral Maxillofac Surg 1997;55:1193–4.

47. Harris M. The conservative management of osteoradionecrosis of the mandible with ultrasound therapy. Br J Oral Maxillofac Surg 1992;30:313–8.

48. Curi MM, Oliveria dos Santos M, Feher O, et al. Management of extensive osteoradionecrosis of the mandible with radical resection and immediate microvascular reconstruction. J Oral Maxillofac Surg 2007;65:434–8.

49. Patuke C, Bauer F, Bissinger O. Tetracycline bone fluorescence: a valuable marker for osteonecrosis characterization and therapy. J Oral Maxillofac Surg 2010;68:125–9.

50. Buchbinder D, Hilaire H. The use of free tissue transfer in advanced osteoradionecrosis of the mandible. J Oral Maxillofac Surg 2006;64:961–4.

51. Bak M, Jacobson AS, Buchbinder D, et al. Contemporary reconstruction of the mandible. Oral Oncol 2010;46:71–6.

52. Suh JD, Blackwell KE, Sercarz JA, et al. Disease relapse after segmental resection and free flap reconstruction for mandibular osteoradionecrosis. Otolaryngol Head Neck Surg 2010;142:586–91.

53. Hidalgo D. Fibula free flap: a new method of mandible reconstruction. Plast Reconstr Surg 1989;84(1):71–9.

54. Jacobson A, Buchbinder D, Urken ML. Reconstruction of bilateral osteoradionecrosis of the mandible using a single fibular free flap. Laryngoscope 2010; 120(2):273.

55. Chaine A, Pitak-Arnnop P, Hivelin M. Postoperative complications of fibular free flaps in mandibular reconstruction: an analysis of 25 consecutive cases. Oral Surg Oral Med Oral Pathol Oral Radiol Endod 2009;108:488–95.

56. Cannady SB, Dean N, Kroeker A, et al. Free flap reconstruction for osteoradionecrosis of the jaws—outcomes and predictive factors for success. Head Neck 2011;33(3):424–8.

57. Wang L, Su YX, Liao GQ. Quality of life in osteoradionecrosis patients after mandible primary reconstruction with free fibula flap. Oral Surg Oral Med Oral Pathol Oral Radiol Endod 2009;108:162–8.

58. Thiel HJ. Osteoradionecrosis. Etiology pathogenesis, clinical aspects and risk factors. Radiobiol Radiother 1989;30:397–413.

Failure to Diagnose Pathology: An Avoidable Complication in Oral and Maxillofacial Surgery

Raymond J. Melrose, DDS[a,b],*

KEYWORDS

• Oral surgery • Maxillofacial surgery • Diagnosis • Pathology

The legal concept of failure to diagnose may assume many forms. The bottom line is, however, that such failure may constitute malpractice. Timely and accurate diagnosis of a medical/dental condition is the first critical step to ensuring appropriate treatment. Each medical/dental practitioner is bound by a legal duty to perform his or her job to a specified standard of care. Whether caused by hurriedness, lack of testing, or a simple mistake, failure to diagnose can constitute a breach of that duty, placing liability for any resulting damages on the medical/dental provider.[1]

Certainly, failure to diagnose oral disease is a leading cause of dental malpractice litigation. Claims of failure to diagnose oral cancer are on the increase.[2] Studdert and colleagues,[3] in a thorough review of *successful* medical malpractice claims, reported that missed or delayed diagnoses represented the grounds for 30% of settled malpractice claims. Only those claims related to surgical misadventures represented a larger proportion of cases (31%). No one is immune from error but the previous information makes it readily apparent that in order to insulate oneself to as great a degree as possible from a significant source of malpractice liability, establishing a definitive diagnosis prior to, or in conjunction with, treatment is of paramount importance.

Several major dental professional organizations have recognized the validity of the previous statement. For example, in 2001, the American Association of Oral and Maxillofacial Surgeons (AAOMS) stated, "evidence-based medicine demonstrates that treatment decisions and their outcomes should be based on a definitive pathologic diagnosis obtained either by preoperative biopsy or post-treatment submission of surgical specimens."[4] The American Association of Endodontists (AAE) said,

A biopsy is appropriate if any of the following conditions exist: (A) When an adequate amount of tissue or foreign material can be removed from the surgical site for histopathologic examination. (B) Persistent pathosis or pathosis inconsistent with endodontic disease is noted on clinical or radiographic examination. (C) Medical history indicates the merits of biopsy.[5]

The American Academy of Oral and Maxillofacial Pathology (AAOMP) recommends that any abnormal tissue removed from patients be submitted promptly for microscopic evaluation and diagnosis, preferably by an oral and maxillofacial pathologist.[6] Further, given the emphasis placed upon the value of evidence-based practice,

[a] Oral Pathology Associates, Inc., 11500 West Olympic Boulevard, Suite 390, Los Angeles, CA 90064, USA
[b] University of Southern California, 925 West 34th Street, Los Angeles, CA 90089, USA
* Oral Pathology Associates, Inc., 11500 West Olympic Boulevard, Suite 390, Los Angeles, CA 90064.
E-mail address: rmelrose@msn.com

Oral Maxillofacial Surg Clin N Am 23 (2011) 465–473
doi:10.1016/j.coms.2011.04.008
1042-3699/11/$ – see front matter © 2011 Elsevier Inc. All rights reserved.

the failure to obtain histologic confirmation of the clinical impression may result in treatment that is only partially evidence based. Clearly then, the advice of major dental professional organizations and simple self-preservation from malpractice litigation strongly support the overarching value of histopathologic diagnosis in patient care.

Of course, virtually all oral and maxillofacial surgeons (OMFS) understand the value of histopathologic diagnosis for difficult or unusual clinical cases or for those in which a malignancy is suspected. But the author's personal experiences over 43 years of practice show that, for various reasons, some OMFS do not routinely submit tissue for examination and report when they think they are reasonably sure of the clinical diagnosis or if patients balk at the extra fee that a pathology report engenders. Often, the surgeon is generally correct in the assessment that a lesion is benign and patients suffer no untoward consequences when the tissue is discarded. Examples of this situation include soft-tissue swellings related to presumed local trauma, such as fibromas and mucoceles; periapical and pericoronal radiolucencies thought to represent apical/periodontal inflammatory disease or dental follicles; leukoplakias of the retromolar region; and lichen planuslike, striated red/white lesions. But this tendency to undervalue a definitive diagnosis that brings the case to complete closure is not only hubris but can lead to trouble if the clinical assessment was incorrect or a recurrence or complication ensues following the surgery. If the in-office procedure had instead been performed in a hospital or surgicenter setting, tissue submission for diagnosis is likely to have been mandatory and to represent the institutional standard of care. Such is not necessarily the case in the private-practice setting, but if it were fewer errors would be made and patients would be better served. A few clinical cases from the records of the author's laboratory illustrate the value of biopsy diagnosis of what seemed to be fairly obvious and straightforward clinical diagnoses (Figs. 1–9).

CASE 1

An adult woman presented with a rubbery, nodular swelling that she had noted for several years. It had not appreciably grown but she sometimes traumatized it during mastication (see **Fig. 1**). The clinical impression was a traumatic fibroma.

- The histopathologic diagnosis was neurofibroma.
- Further examination and workup disclosed several cutaneous nodules that were diagnosed as neurofibromas. She was found

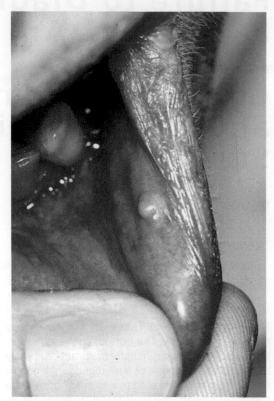

Fig. 1. Rubbery, nodular swelling present without change for several years.

to carry the NF1 gene and 2 of her 3 children were also diagnosed with neurofibromatosis as a result.

Lesson

The value of the histopathologic diagnosis in this case lies in the subsequent evaluations that determined that the family carried the NF1 gene with attendant implications for genetic counseling.

CASE 2

An adult woman was noted to have an asymptomatic periapical radiolucency on tooth #19 (see **Fig. 2**). Tooth-vitality testing was equivocal. The clinical impression was a periapical inflammatory process/apical cyst.

- The histopathologic diagnosis was a metastatic adenocarcinoma.
- When the diagnosis was given to the patient, she revealed that she had recently been diagnosed with breast cancer. The metastatic disease was microscopically similar in all respects to the breast carcinoma.

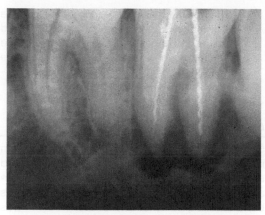

Fig. 2. Asymptomatic periapical radiolucency tooth #19. Vitality testing was equivocal.

Lesson

In addition to the fact that patients do not always provide full disclosure of important medical information to dentists or other health care providers, the tissue diagnosis changed the clinical stage in which the patient was placed and, thus, may have altered the treatment options being considered.

CASE 3

An adult man presented with an extensive reticular-like leukoplakia of the buccal mucosa associated with an erythematous background (see **Fig. 3**). This leukoplakia was sensitive to spicy foods and had been noted for approximately 2 months. There was no history of tobacco use. The clinical impression was lichen planus.

- The histopathologic diagnosis was intense lichenoid mucositis.

- When the diagnosis was received, the patient's chart was reviewed again and it was noted that he had been taking a prescription nonsteroidal antiinflammatory drug for tennis elbow for approximately 6 months. The drug was among those associated with oral lichenoid reactions. When the drug was withdrawn, the lesions slowly resolved over the course of 2 months without additional treatment.

Lesson

Lichenoid reactions should always be considered in the differential diagnosis of clinical findings that suggest lichen planus. Only a well-made biopsy can distinguish between the two, and on some occasions immunofluorescence microscopy may also be required. Further, oral lichenoid reactions are common and do not satisfactorily respond to treatment commonly prescribed for symptomatic lichen planus. As in the previous instance, the identification of a food, medication, or restorative material hypersensitivity may clear the problem when the allergen is withdrawn or is replaced by a nonallergenic substance.

CASE 4

An adult man was referred for evaluation of an asymptomatic leukoplakia in the midline of the palate (see **Fig. 4**). He did not smoke. The clinical impression was a keratosis but the site and presentation were unusual. Biopsy was recommended, but the patient declined because he did not wish to incur the additional expense and was content just to have the abnormality removed. When he was told that the differential diagnosis included

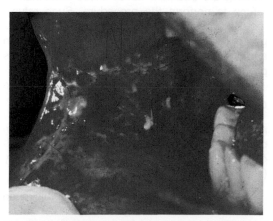

Fig. 3. Erythematous, reticular lesion present for 2 months and sensitive to spicy foods.

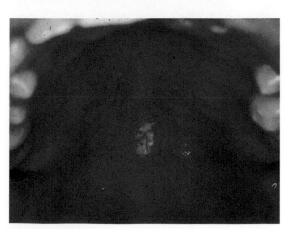

Fig. 4. Asymptomatic, demarcated leukoplakia in midline hard palate.

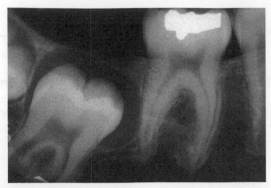

Fig. 5. Demarcated, unilocular pericoronal radiolucency of tooth #18 in a 13-year-old child. Note angle between the mesial cervical line and the edge of the radiolucency.

epithelial dysplasia, and this was explained to him as a premalignant process, he relented.

- The histopathologic diagnosis was bowenoid papulosis.
- Bowenoid papulosis is a human papillomavirus–related condition that is typically acquired by sexual transmission. It is rare in the oral cavity. It has worrisome microscopic

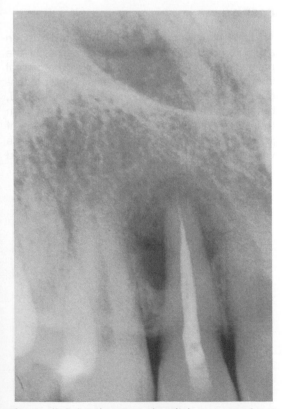

Fig. 6. Ill-defined periapical radiolucency persistent after nonsurgical endodontic treatment.

features but there is as yet no clear evidence that it presents patients with an increased risk of oral cancer.[7] When the nature of the condition was explained to the patient, he admitted that he was engaging in promiscuous oral sex with both genders.

Lesson

Of course this patient is putting himself at an increased risk of other sexually transmitted diseases that may have serious consequences and this knowledge may serve to alter his behavior. But, for the OMFS the problem was convincing the patient that the extra cost of the histopathologic examination was necessary. Most times patients will accept the OMFS recommendation for microscopic examination of biopsied tissue, but there are other times when patients will resist the recommendation. In the previous vignette, the clinical differential diagnosis did include a premalignant condition and the patient accepted. But, if the patient continued to decline, would the OMFS be absolved from risk of failure to diagnose if the diagnosis had been that of a premalignant condition and the patient subsequently developed a carcinoma and brought suit? There is not a definitive answer to that question. Can patients really sign an informed consent that declares his or her refusal to accept a professional recommendation and lose the right to sue or recover damages? Again, one would wish that it were so but nothing is sure, especially when a jury is involved. In the author's view, the best protection is to not let patients make important medical decisions, such as whether a histopathologic examination of abnormal tissue is needed or justified. Certainly, an OMFS would not let patients dictate which instruments to use in a procedure. If patients are adamant about tissue examination, refuse to perform the procedure. Such refusal may often be the trigger that changes the patients' perception about the necessity of the examination and then the OMFS can bring the case to its proper conclusion with a definitive diagnosis.

CASE 5

A 13-year-old child presents with delayed eruption of tooth #18. The radiograph showed a well-demarcated, unilocular pericoronal radiolucency (see **Fig. 5**).

- The clinical impression was thickened follicle versus dentigerous cyst.
- The histopathologic diagnosis was unicystic ameloblastoma.

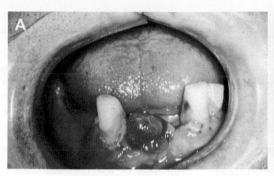
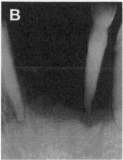

Fig. 7. (*A*) Painless mass developed after patient self-extracted several loose mandibular incisors. (*B*) Bone loss and a floating bone spicule.

- There was no evidence of growth into the wall (mural extension) or of transmural growth in the enucleated specimen, so no additional therapy was performed. There was no recurrence.

Lesson

Many OMFS do not routinely submit follicles of impacted teeth even if there is some suggestion that a dentigerous cyst might be present in the form of a thickness more than 5 mm or an angle between the cervical line of the tooth and the edge of the radiolucency that is 45° or greater (note the angle on the mesial aspect of the impacted tooth in the illustration). This risk should not be taken. The differential diagnosis of a lesion such as just described includes not only the 2 conditions considered by the clinician but the actual diagnosis and an odontogenic keratocyst (OKC). Certainly, if a dentigerous cyst is in the differential, then OKC and unicystic ameloblastoma should be. The risk of recurrence of OKC and of unicystic ameloblastoma is high compared to that of a dentigerous cyst. About the only things protecting OMFS who do not routinely submit peri-follicular tissues for histopathologic examination when a dentigerous cyst is in the differential from untoward consequences are odds and luck and luck is fickle.

CASE 6

An adult man had previous nonsurgical endodontics performed by another dentist. When a periapical radiolucency failed to resolve, he referred the patient to an endodontist for apicoectomy (see **Fig. 6**).

- The clinical impression was apical cyst/granuloma.
- The histopathologic diagnosis was odontogenic myxoma.

Lesson

The endodontist is one who routinely submits periapical tissues for histopathologic examination as per the recommendation of the AAE. This diagnosis was the first surprise diagnosis he had received, although he has been practicing for 11 years. No one likes to receive unpleasant surprises, but if the tissue had not been submitted, this infiltrating odontogenic neoplasm would have continued to grow and when the correct diagnosis was finally achieved, the endodontist could have been in a difficult situation to defend if the patient had become angry or was advised to take action. The prudent course of action for all surgeons, in the author's view, is to routinely submit all abnormal tissues removed as per the recommendations of AAOMS, AAE and AAOMP (with the exceptions of carious teeth, impacted teeth without enlarged follicles, gingiva removed for pocket reduction, excess tissue following mucosal plastic procedures, and known foreign material).

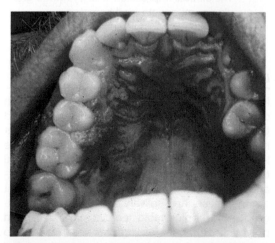

Fig. 8. Second recurrence of a gingival mass following curettage and tissue discarding by a general dentist.

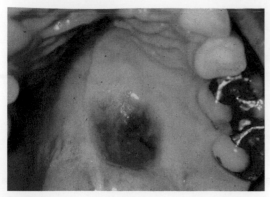

Fig. 9. Red, tender swelling thought to have developed following trauma by a chicken bone sliver.

CASE 7

An elderly man with advanced periodontal disease presented to an OMFS complaining of a bleeding, painless growth at the site where 2 lower incisors had been recently self-extracted because they were so loose (see **Fig. 7**A). Radiograph showed the bone loss and a bone spicule (see **Fig. 7**B).

- The clinical impression was pyogenic granuloma.
- The histopathologic diagnosis was squamous cell carcinoma of the gingiva.

Lesson

Gingival squamous cell carcinomas may simulate advanced periodontal disease, and this possibility should always be considered when or if conventional treatment for the periodontal problem fails to resolve the situation or, as in this case, extraction is followed by a rapidly growing soft-tissue mass. When a tooth or teeth are extracted from the site of a carcinoma, the increased blood supply to the wound may dramatically accelerate tumor growth.

CASE 8

This adult man was referred to an OMFS by a general dentist for re-removal of hyperplastic-appearing tissue that had been removed by curettage on 2 previous occasions (see **Fig. 8**). The dentist had discarded the tissues each time thinking they were some form of reactive process, such as a pyogenic granuloma. The OMFS thought that a diagnosis of pyogenic granuloma might be correct but was hard pressed to determine a reason for it. When he advised the dentist of his intention to send the tissues for histopathologic examination, the dentist objected. The OMFS

refused to perform the procedure unless biopsy confirmation of the diagnosis was the result and the dentist acceded.

- The clinical impression was gingival reactive process/rule out cancer.
- The histopathologic diagnosis was malignant amelanotic melanoma.

Lesson

Apropos of the previous case, it is clear that gingival reactive processes may simulate cancer clinically and vice versa. The actual diagnosis was a devastating one for the patient and the doctors alike. The OMFS was not convinced of the likelihood of a reactive process because he could not see a good reason for it even though the teeth were slightly misaligned. Reactive processes in the oral cavity are among the most common histopathologic diagnoses made by oral pathologists, and some surgeons are dubious of the value of histopathologic confirmation of such a common group of lesions. However, reactive lesions have a high recurrence rate if the local causative factors are not addressed, and without a definitive diagnosis in the chart, there is always concern that an error in clinical evaluation might have occurred if the lesion recurs. Knowing the correct diagnosis should give the surgeon considerable peace of mind when dealing with an unexpected recurrence.

CASE 9

An adult woman developed a tender swelling shortly after traumatizing the palate with a sliver of a chicken bone (see **Fig. 9**).

- The clinical impression was pyogenic granuloma, mucocele, and hematoma.
- The histopathologic diagnosis was low-grade mucoepidermoid carcinoma.

Lesson

Mucoceles of the hard palate are uncommon despite the abundance of minor salivary gland tissue there. As a general rule, lesions that resemble mucoceles in locations other than the lower lip, buccal mucosa, and anterior ventral tongue should have other diagnostic considerations placed higher than a mucocele. Frequent among these are salivary gland tumors. Low-grade mucoepidermoid carcinomas are often polycystic, thus, increasing their resemblance to a mucocele, a vascular tumor, or a pigmented lesion. In this instance, the OMFS waited several weeks to observe resolution if the swelling represented a hematoma. When it did not change, the biopsy was immediately performed.

A surgeon should always perform a biopsy of abnormal tissue if the differential diagnosis includes even 1 significant entity. Thus, a differential diagnosis of even the most mundane or common-appearing lesions should be made and entered into the patient record. Clearly, OMFS have excellent training and experience in oral pathology and their clinical impression (defined as the most likely possibility in the differential diagnostic list) of an abnormality should, in most cases, be correct. But, as the previous examples have shown, no one is always correct. Frankly, even the best clinical diagnosis is an educated guess until confirmation of that diagnosis has been received. The confirmation may be in the form of supplemental testing, such as culture and sensitivity; additional or special radiographs; or tissue examination. But the important point here is that confirmation should be sought. Just anticipating that a surgically removed lesion will not recur may seem to be expedient but it will not confirm that a clinical impression is accurate. Patients are entitled to our most accurate diagnosis because accurate diagnosis is the cornerstone of appropriate treatment.

According to a recent publication by Raab and Grzybicki,[8] approximately 1.6 million patients in the United States will be diagnosed with cancer in 2010. Many millions more will have tissue samples obtained to rule out cancer but who do not have that disease. With so many positive and negative tissue samples being evaluated annually, diagnostic error becomes an important issue. The reported frequency of diagnostic error made by oncologic pathology depends on several factors, such as definitions and detection methods and ranges from 1% to 15%. According to these same investigators, the large majority of diagnostic errors do not result in severe harm, although mild to moderate harm in the form of additional testing or diagnostic delay occurs in up to 50% of cases. These investigators conclude that clinical practitioners play an essential role in error reduction through several avenues, such as effective test ordering, providing accurate and pertinent clinical information, procuring high-quality specimens, providing timely follow-up on test results, effectively communicating on potentially discrepant diagnoses, and advocating second opinions on the pathology diagnosis in specific situations. Because parts of what has been previously stated regarding oncologic testing may be equally true for the more common situation of routine biopsy by an oral and maxillofacial surgeon, the author addresses specific ways to improve the diagnostic process when the decision to perform a biopsy has already been made. The author calls these items the "methods for optimum results" and they include the following topics: proper site selection; removal of sufficient tissue; avoidance of artifact; proper and adequate fixation; correct identification of the specimens; adequate, accurate history with radiographs, as appropriate; legible, complete paperwork; avoiding delay in sample submission; and correlation of the diagnosis received with the clinical impression.

1. Biopsy site selection: For a planned excisional biopsy, this should not be a problem. For an incisional biopsy, however, it may be critical. First, it must be understood that an incisional biopsy is performed for a single purpose: to obtain a definitive diagnosis upon which any further needed treatment may be based. With that purpose in mind, one should try to include in the specimen as much tissue representative of the disease process as possible. The old dictum that a biopsy should always include a margin of normal may interfere with that objective and is often not necessary. A margin of normal tissue is valuable when assessing sloughing or vesiculating diseases and ulcers, but in most other situations does not add value to the process and may interfere with accuracy if too much normal and too little disease is provided. One should not hesitate to submit more than 1 specimen from a large lesion or when a single incisional specimen cannot include all the different clinical features of significance.

2. Removal of sufficient tissue is clearly important. As a general rule, small lesions should be excised. For incisional biopsies, provide the pathologist with as large a specimen as possible consistent with the patients' postoperative comfort and the ability to close the wound. Tiny specimens may inhibit accurate embedding of the sample in the paraffin block and may impair the pathologist's ability to provide an unequivocal diagnosis. When it is important for the pathologist to comment on margins for adequacy of excision, the margins should be clearly labeled by the surgeon. Using 1 or more sutures is a simple method of distinguishing margins in excised specimens. Incisional biopsy of swellings, such as a suspected salivary gland tumor, should take into account that a deep biopsy is often more likely to be representative than a shallow one because these tumors may develop deep and push normal tissues ahead. Fine-needle aspiration biopsy (FNA) has become a valuable adjunct in management of tumorlike masses in sites, such as the breast, thyroid gland, parotid gland, and prostate gland,

because open biopsy of these sites brings on complications that FNA may avoid. But there are few oral masses that are subject to these complications of site. Although FNA has proven to be valuable, it is not as accurate as a tissue sample and is not preferred for assessment of lesions accessible by a knife. Biopsy of solid bony lesions may be challenging, but trephine instruments, such as those now used routinely for coring out bone for implant placement, may be excellent tools to obtain a representative piece while maintaining important physical relationships between cortical surfaces and deeper tissues.

3. Avoidance of artifact: Careful tissue handling is important. Grasping or pulling on tissue with forceps may be convenient, but forceps compression or use of a toothed forceps may induce tearing and other artifacts that may interfere with interpretation. The simple use of a suture placed through a specimen prior to removal facilitates specimen control and avoids artifact. It is usually preferable to use a sharp cutting instrument rather than one that produces heat, such as with a laser or cauterizing instrument, to remove a sample. This point is particularly so if the lesion is small. Heat induces serious artifact that may interfere with diagnosis or compromise the assessment of margins. Similarly, avoid the use of solutions that stain the surface, such as iodine-type solutions. The usual marking pens and toluidine blue, on the other hand, do not interfere with staining or interpretation.

4. Immediate and proper fixation: Fixation is imperative to avoid autolysis of tissues. As soon as the specimen is free, it should be placed in the fixative material supplied by the laboratory. The most common fixative in use today is formalin. Other fixatives may be needed for specific functions, such as immunofluorescence, but these will also be provided. A formalin-fixed specimen cannot be used for immunofluorescence, so the need for that technique must be determined in advance. Never alter, dilute, or in any other way change the fixative provided unless specific instructions for that procedure are given in advance. Remember also that formalin is an aqueous solution of formaldehyde that is dilute and has been buffered to neutral pH. Prolonged storage may cause evaporation of water or precipitation of buffering chemicals. It is best to rotate formalin containers such that the oldest are used first. Formaldehyde is considered to be a toxin and a carcinogenic substance when used inappropriately or in large volumes over prolonged periods, but it has little harmful potential in the small amounts typically placed in specimen containers. However, bottles should remain tightly closed until use and then tightly closed again for shipment to the laboratory. Be sure to follow the directions given by the laboratory for safe shipment via the US Postal Service or other carrier.

5. Proper specimen identification: When more than 1 specimen is submitted from patients, these must each be clearly identified as to site. Placing a suture in one and not the other is a convenient method, but be sure to indicate which is which on the request sheet. Separate bottles need not be used if that precaution is followed. To rely on differences in specimen size, shape, or color to distinguish one biopsy site from another may not be wise. Fixed tissue shrinks, may become distorted, and changes color. Certainly, the anatomic location of the biopsy specimens must be given to the laboratory on the biopsy request form in order to be recorded on the report. This idea seems intuitive, but it is amazing how often this simple but important step is mishandled.

6. Submit an adequate, accurate history with radiographs as appropriate. Examining a piece of tissue under a microscope is not a task that should be done in isolation. To properly diagnose a specimen, the oral pathologist may need to review the history and the clinical setting in which the patients' condition manifested. Indeed, sometimes this information is absolutely critical. Radiographic evaluation and correlation with histopathologic findings may be indispensable in accurate diagnosis. Images provided as copies, originals, on CDs, or in e-mails are all valuable. The author prefers not to give a definitive diagnosis of many osseous lesions without having assessed the images personally or at least read a cogent written description or interpretation by the submitting surgeon.

7. Submit legible and complete paperwork. Legibility speaks for itself. Complete and accurate paperwork means that the doctor or a designated, responsible staff person has ensured that all requested information has been provided. To do less may mean delay in processing and delay in diagnosis. The information requested is not superfluous; it is mandated by federal and state laws and regulations that patients and their tissues be uniquely identifiable to the greatest degree possible, consistent with Health Insurance Portability and Accountability Act requirements. This practice is not an intrusion on privacy; rather, it is for patient protection. All information provided as history is treated with similar discretion.

8. Forward the specimen promptly. The laboratory will provide a means for sending the sample. Tissues fixed in formalin may be kept in diagnosable condition for some time, but never delay sending the sample because that will delay diagnosis. Recently, in conversations with other oral pathologists, we have learned that, for reasons known only to themselves, some doctors are removing tissues but not sending them immediately for diagnosis. Instead, the tissues in the formalin-filled bottles are retained until such time as the lesion in question recurs or some untoward circumstance develops. Then the tissues are submitted. The author is not an attorney, but thinks that a lawyer would have a field day with such behavior in a failure-to-diagnose malpractice action.

9. Always correlate the diagnosis provided with the clinical impression. Although the author placed this last simply from a sequencing standpoint, it is probably one of the most important steps in the entire process. Clearly, most clinical diagnoses are going to be accurate as to the basic disease process. The specific diagnosis may be at slight variance with the clinical impression, but if the variance does not impact treatment or prognosis in any significant way, it may be considered to be accurate and no more action may be needed. On the other hand, if the histopathologic diagnosis is at a significant variance with the clinical impression, then something more will need to be done to verify which is more accurate. Pathologists may make errors in interpretation, specimens may have been mislabeled, and there are other possibilities for variance. But it is the clinician responsible for the patients' care who must initiate action. A telephone call to the pathologist may uncover a laboratory error. If there is no laboratory error, a second opinion may be needed. If the biopsy was inadequate for some reason, the pathologist should articulate that to the surgeon. But the single most important point is that the patients' best interests and welfare are paramount.

In summary, the routine submission of abnormal tissue for histopathologic diagnosis is a vital link in the appropriate management of patients. Receipt of a biopsy report brings the usual case to its full conclusion. Patients are best served when clinical impressions are verified by histopathologic examination, and this, in turn, will reduce the likelihood of successful malpractice litigation for failure or delay in diagnosis.

REFERENCES

1. Failure to diagnose: medical malpractice. Available at: http://www.medicalmalprctice.com. Accessed April 27, 2010.
2. Raap C. Oral cancer malpractice claims increasing. Todays FDA 2005;17:37–8.
3. Studdert DM, Mello MM, Gawande AA, et al. Claims, errors and compensation payments in medical malpractice litigation. N Engl J Med 2006;354: 2024–33.
4. Parameters and pathways: clinical practice guidelines for oral and maxillofacial surgery; diagnosis and management of pathologic conditions. Chicago: American Association of Oral and Maxillofacial Surgeons; 2001.
5. Guide to clinical endodontics. Chicago: American Association of Endodontists; 2004.
6. Submission policy on excised tissue. Available at: http://www.aaomp.org/home/healthcareprofessionals. Accessed October 12, 2010.
7. Rinaggio J, Glick M, Lambert WC. Oral bowenoid papulosis in an HIV-positive male. Oral Surg Oral Med Oral Pathol Oral Radiol Endod 2006;101:328–32.
8. Raab SS, Grzybicki DM. Quality in cancer diagnosis. CA Cancer J Clin 2010;60:139–65.

The Law and Dentoalveolar Complications: Trends and Controversies

Arthur W. Curley, JD[a,b,*]

KEYWORDS

- Maxillofacial surgery • Standard of care • Informed consent
- Risk management

OVERVIEW

Despite appropriate planning, execution, and follow-up, patients can and do experience complications from oral and maxillofacial surgical procedures. The occurrence of a complication is often unpredictable, which is one of the reasons that oral and maxillofacial surgery is often described as much an art as a science.

However, the occurrence of postoperative complications in some situations can trigger claims of substandard care. This article reviews the legal standards associated with complications, provides case studies, and makes recommendations to avoid such claims.

LEGAL PRINCIPLES

A review of the legal principles associated with claims of malpractice in oral surgery is essential to understanding the legal issues associated with complications.

With few exceptions, oral surgery malpractice laws are determined by the individual state in which the surgery is performed. The inherent limits of space in this article as well as their purpose, prevent the listing of the specific laws of all 50 states, Washington, DC, and the territory of Puerto Rico. General references can be found on the Internet (see http://www.mcandl.com/states.html).

All states adhere to a few basic principles. An oral surgery malpractice claim requires the proof of three basic elements of Tort Law: negligence, cause, and injury. Professional negligence is generally defined as failure to meet or adhere to the standard of care.

THE LAW AND THE STANDARD OF CARE

During the education and training of an oral and maxillofacial surgeon, the practitioner is taught standards of care for diagnosis and treatment. Thereafter, the oral surgery standard of care is set by the community of clinicians trained and licensed to perform oral and maxillofacial surgery. However, the legal standard of care can be broader and more dynamic. The law can create standards by legislation, rule, or regulation, regardless of the prevailing surgical standard of care. For example, one generally-accepted standard of care is to educate patients regarding a proposed treatment, such as IV sedation, and obtain the patient's consent, known as informed consent. That is a surgical standard of care. Risk management principles recommend the use of written documentation for most informed consents. However, in some states, such as California, by statute, all dentists must obtain written informed consent before performing IV sedation (California Business and Professions Code 1682e). The prudent practitioner, hoping to avoid being drawn into the legal system, should have an appreciation of the legal as well as the surgical standards of care and associated

a Arthur A. Dugoni School of Dentistry, University of the Pacific, San Francisco, CA, USA
b Bradley, Curley, Asiano, Barrabee, Abel & Kowalski, P.C., Larkspur, CA, USA
* Arthur A. Dugoni School of Dentistry, University of the Pacific, San Francisco, CA.
E-mail address: acurley@professionals-law.com

Oral Maxillofacial Surg Clin N Am 23 (2011) 475–484
doi:10.1016/j.coms.2011.04.003

doctrines, and implement that knowledge in practice protocols.

Legal, rather than community, standards of care are determined by the written laws (statutes) of the state in which the dental professional practices and is licensed. For example, not all states require written informed consent for IV sedation. Until recently, not all states required a permit for IV sedation. However, these laws are seldom specific to any method of diagnosis, plan, or required treatment. Rather, the laws are general with regard to the definition of the community legal standards of care. In addition, there are Federal laws that can affect the practice of surgery, such as the Health Insurance Portability and Accountability Act (HIPAA) and the Occupational Safety and Health Act (OSHA).[1,2]

The law defines the community standard of care as follows: "A surgeon is negligent if he/she fails to exercise the level of skill, knowledge, and care in diagnosis and treatment that other reasonably careful surgeons would possess and use in the same or similar circumstances. This level of skill, knowledge and care is generally referred to as 'the standard of care'."[3] The legal standard of care is not limited to the very best care or to treatment by only the best surgeon. Nor is it the average care in the community. It is that minimum level of care to which a patient is entitled, as described in testimony by expert witnesses.

Failure to provide treatment that meets the standard of care is considered professional negligence or what is commonly referred to as malpractice. To prevail in a malpractice claim, the patient must prove four elements: (1) that the surgeon owed a duty to the patient; (2) that the surgeon failed to meet the legal standard of care; (3) that the failure was the legal cause; and (4) an injury. Only after proving these four elements can a jury or court award damages (money) to a patient.[4]

Attorneys cannot, and therefore do not, determine the standard of care. The community standard of care is determined by the opinion of expert witnesses testifying in court or before an administrative law judge in a dental board accusation. The standard of care against which the acts of a surgeon are to be measured is a matter peculiarly within the knowledge of experts. It presents the basic issue in a malpractice action and can only be proved by their expert testimony, unless the conduct required by the particular circumstances is within the common knowledge of the layman.[5] For example, as to the standard of care to be applied to a claim of anesthesia injury, expert testimony is required because of the complexity of the issues. By comparison, in a claim alleging extraction of the wrong tooth, expert witness testimony would not be required as to issues of the standard of care, but would still be required as to the issues associated with the appropriate method and costs to replace the wrongfully-removed tooth.

In a malpractice suit, a jury of mostly lay persons determines whether or not a surgeon violated the standard of care by comparing and contrasting the evidence provided by each side (plaintiff vs defendant) in a trial. They hear testimony from expert witnesses and view radiographs and records.

The legal qualifications for an expert witness include being licensed to perform the treatment in question or having expertise in one of the issues in dispute, such as standards of care for implants or the cause of a particular injury (eg, a postoperative infection). An expert may be a general practitioner or a specialist in the area of the treatment in question. The law in most states does not require an expert to have the identical training or certification of the defendant, although Arizona requires matching certification. While not common, a general dentist can testify against a board-certified specialist or vice versa in most states but with little credibility. Courts typically rule that credentials and board certification merely support the credibility of an expert and that the jury or judge may weigh in determining whom to believe. Juries may evaluate expert witnesses on their style or mannerisms, in addition to whether their statements seem to be supported by the other evidence in the case, such as imaging, records, or published studies.

Juries may discount the testimony of board-certified dental specialists who are also professors and authors in favor of a general dentist who testifies in a simple, logical fashion and renders easy-to-understand opinions that make common sense and are supported by the evidence. Therefore, maintaining clear and reasonably detailed records regarding oral and maxillofacial care is essential in avoiding claims of substandard care. An expert witness may also testify on issues of causation without having to render opinion as to the standard of care or without even having had training in surgery. For example, in cases of bacterial endocarditis, the law will allow testimony from an expert in heart valves or postoperative infections, such as a cardiologist or an infectious disease physician.

Expert witnesses typically come from two sources: treating surgeons and retained experts.[6] Often they are subsequent care providers who have expressed some criticisms of the care given by another surgeon or attributed the cause of some injury to prior dental care or the lack thereof (ie, failure to diagnose postoperative fracture).

Such experts are called nonretained expert witnesses.[7] Other expert witnesses are those who may not have seen the patient for treatment but are hired by the attorney for either the plaintiff or the defendant to evaluate the standard of care and/or causation by reviewing records, imaging, testimony, and sometimes by examining the patient. Such experts are called retained expert witnesses.[8] Whereas, nonretained experts are only paid for the time spent giving testimony, retained experts are typically paid for the time spent reviewing the evidence in the case in addition to time spent in testimony. The practical reality is that each party to a malpractice suit will hire experts with a proclivity to their side of the case: pro-patient versus pro-practitioner.

Although the law allows an expert to be both a treating health care provider and a retained expert witness, in some states it may be considered unethical and a conflict of interest.[9] The conflict issue stems from the potential that a subsequent treating surgeon may provide a patient with a treatment plan, such as the placement of several implants, and then provide testimony that the plan was necessitated by the previous treatment of the defendant, because in the expert's opinion it was less than the standard of care. Such ethical violations, although admissible evidence in trial to challenge the credibility of the expert witness, are not per se a violation of a statute and, therefore, will not cause the court to exclude the witness.

Experts can also render opinion as to the management of dental auxiliaries, such as surgical assistants, and their impact on the surgeon's ability to perform within the standard of care. Examples include negligent transmission of referral information, failure to schedule follow-up appointments or recalls, failure to maintain OSHA standards, or failure to follow safety protocols in radiography. This rule of law is called respondeat superior, meaning that an employer surgeon or dental corporation is vicariously liable for the wrongful acts of its employees, committed when they were acting within the scope of their employment, even if they violated office rules or protocols. Equally well established is the principle that an employee's willful, malicious, or even criminal acts may be within the scope of employment for purposes of respondeat superior, even though the employer had not authorized the employee to commit crimes or intentional wrongful acts.[10] For example, an employee charged with collections gets into a heated argument with a patient and pushes that person, who then falls backward over a chair and is seriously injured. The employer is liable for that injury because the employee was performing, albeit poorly, within the scope of his/her job duties in trying to collect overdue funds. The prudent practitioner should establish protocols to promote staff compliance with standards of care and conduct routine audits to evaluate compliance. Use of specific checklists for various tasks is helpful for training and auditing staff.

WRITTEN STANDARDS OF CARE

Expert witnesses may bolster their opinions by the use of authoritative or well-recognized texts, peer-reviewed journals, or treatises. However, whether a text is considered authoritative or well-recognized is determined by a judge, who considers expert witness testimony as to the qualifications of the text or journal on an issue before it can be read to a jury.[10] Guidelines, such as those of the American Heart Association, are documents that also may be considered evidence of the standard of care.[11]

Written guidelines can be used as a standard of care if they were so intended by the authors. The guidelines of the American Society of Anesthesiologists (ASA) were intended to set standards of care to reduce mobility and mortality.[12] These guidelines are part of the typical oral and maxillofacial residency program. Also, the ASA guidelines may be admitted in most courts as evidence of standards of care for anesthesia. Therefore, most surgeons providing anesthesia follow those guidelines. For example, failure to rate a patient as ASA 1 to 4 may be evidence of substandard care in the event of an anesthesia complication.

On the other hand, the parameters of care of the American Society of Oral & Maxillofacial Surgeons are specifically meant not to be standards of care; however, some courts have allowed their admission as evidence.[13]

Surgical technologies, such as dental implants, come with manufacturer's guidelines. Although not specifically stated or intended as setting standards of care, courts commonly allow experts to testify that a defendant's failure to adhere to the manufacturer's guidelines, such as the specific use of a pilot drill, was a violation of the standard of care.

WRITTEN LAWS: CODE

In most states, the violation of a statute that is designed and intended to prevent harm (such as failure to autoclave surgical instruments) is presumptive evidence of a violation of the standard of care or professional negligence, and, in such cases, expert testimony is not required. A typical case might be the failure to adhere to OSHA regulations for the management of potential blood-borne pathogens. For example, should a patient develop a postsurgical infection, ordinarily a known risk of any surgery, evidence of an OSHA blood-borne pathogens standards violation would be considered evidence of substandard care, and the defendant's only defense would be to prove the lack of a causation of the infection by the OSHA violation. In such a case, expert testimony would not be required on the issue of a breach of the standard of care. However, expert testimony may still be required as to causation; ie, did the statutory violation cause the infection?

DAMAGES

In the event of the finding by a jury or court of a breach of the standard of care that caused an injury, the patient can recover two types of damages: general and special. General damages are for physical and emotional pain and suffering. Special damages are for financial losses, such as medical bills, wages, and traveling expenses. Therefore, it is important to note and chart the details and specifics of a patient's postsurgical complaints and track their course. For example, when a patient suffers from residual numbness after an extraction or implant placement, the course of the injury and, therefore, damages should be charted with specifics and details at subsequent examinations.[14] In addition, risk management dictates that postsurgical examinations should also include notation of the absence of neurologic or other complications. That way, if the patient should develop subsequent symptoms, the cause can be better understood or the patient's credibility challenged. In the case of numbness after an extraction or placement of an implant, the onset and degree of numbness may indicate the cause and even effect of whether or not a claim for malpractice is made.

COMPARATIVE FAULT/CONTRIBUTORY NEGLIGENCE

The law of negligence provides that if a patient is also negligent, such as failing to take antibiotics as instructed, his/her claim for malpractice may be reduced or even defeated. Most states follow the rule of comparative fault, meaning that the negligence of the patient merely reduces the amount of the damages that will be awarded by his/her percentage of fault.[15] A few states follow the doctrine of contributory negligence, which means that if the patient is at fault to any degree, their claim for malpractice will be extinguished.[16] Therefore, it is essential to note and chart whenever a patient misses an appointment, fails to follow instructions, or provides a false or deceptive history.

BURDEN OF PROOF

In a typical malpractice case, the patient's attorney has the burden of proving a violation of the standard of care, but unlike criminal cases where the evidentiary level is beyond a reasonable doubt, the plaintiff in a malpractice case need only provide evidence of a probability (not a certainty) of a breach of the standard of care. This is called a preponderance of the evidence. A probability in law means greater than 50%, meaning that a jury can have 49% doubt and still find that the defendant failed to meet the standard of care.[17] Because of the reduced level of evidence required in a malpractice case compared with a criminal case, the surgeon should be vigilant in keeping records and documenting consultations with other health care providers as well as with the patient. It has been the trial experience of this author that in resolving conflicting testimony between a patient and a surgeon, juries favor the surgeon's testimony when it is supported by detailed and legible documentation.

As a cautionary note, records should be kept in the ordinary course of treatment and not amended in response to a patient filing a suit, complaint, or even a threat by the patient. Alteration of records may significantly damage a dental care provider's credibility and lead to a separate claim of alteration of evidence to deceive.[18]

INFORMED CONSENT

The laws of most states require that surgeons obtain informed consent before providing treatment.[19] A surgeon is required to disclose all information relevant to a meaningful decision process and obtain the fully-informed consent of the patient or the patient's legal guardian before treatment. If imaging or models are used as part of the consent process, that fact should be charted and the object or educational tool identified. The laws are not specific as to the details that must be part of the informed consent discussion, and only require that the patient be told the significant risks, benefits, and alternatives to recommended treatments, therapies, or medications.

With a few exceptions (eg, IV sedation: California Code of Regulations, Section 1685), the law does not require that the informed consent be in writing. However, written documentation is a deterrent to claims of lack of informed consent. Studies have shown that patients do not recall pretreatment discussions, and they can insist with credibility that they were not warned.[20]

INFORMED REFUSAL

Surgery has become more technical and complex, providing more treatment options for patients, and resulting in new exposure potential. The obligation to obtain informed refusal or explaining the risks of declining a recommended treatment, therapy, or medication must be documented. When a patient refuses to accept recommended or ideal treatment or advice (eg, because of costs), the prudent surgeon should obtain and document informed refusal.[21] This is known as documenting the discussion of the risks, benefits, and alternatives to refusing recommended treatment or selecting a less than ideal treatment plan.

A simple chart note can be effective documentation of an informed refusal discussion. For example, in a case where a patient is advised to have an impacted molar removed and, despite discussing the risks of not going forward, the patient declines, the following chart note can be made and then signed by the patient: "[Patient Name] advised of need to remove #16; Patient refuses. Risks, benefits, and alternatives discussed, including the potential for infection and injury to #15. Patient still declines. [X Patient Signature]." By having the patient read and sign a chart entry that notes that they were advised of the worst risks of refusal (in this case, infection) and still declined, the law assumes the patient would have declined had they been told of any lesser risks. In the case of electronic records, the patient can either sign a digital pad as used today for credit card purchases, or the form can be printed, signed, and scanned back to the e-file as a PDF file.

STANDARD OF CARE FOR REFERRALS

Another legal standard is the duty to refer for treatment. Although most often applied to general dentists, the standard also applies to specialists, such as oral and maxillofacial surgeons. Most state laws merely say that it is necessary to refer when it would be reasonable to do so without specific guidelines.

The following tenets are typically used by expert witnesses testifying for the plaintiff. Whether a patient can be treated or needs to be referred to another specialist is determined by whether the surgeon can: (1) predict the potential for complications and, therefore, by prepared for them (such as having resuscitation equipment at the ready and the experience to use it); (2) recognize the occurrence of a complication in timely fashion and initiate appropriate treatment (such as recognizing the absence of breath sounds and beginning basic life support); (3) recognize the occurrence of a complication and make a timely referral (such as calling 911 at the onset of respiratory failure).

DOCUMENTING MEDICAL CONSULTATIONS

The patient's medical history may indicate the need for medical clearance to perform oral and maxillofacial surgery. Ideally, the surgeon should obtain a signed clearance from the appropriate health care provider. However, there are occasions where only verbal clearance can be obtained.

Tips

Documentation of a telephonic medical clearance can be made by way of a confirming fax (**Figs. 1** and **2**, **Box 1**). In most states, courts recognize that confirming fax letters can be used as evidence of the terms of a conversation, if not denied by the recipient within 2 to 3 business days of transmission.[22] Proof is obtained by sending the fax via a machine that will produce an activity report after each transmission. The report can be designed to include a copy of the transmission as well as the date, time, number, and indication of successful or failed transmission. This report, if successfully transmitted, should be added to the patient's chart and the original need not be mailed.

Complications

All surgical procedures have risks of complications that can and do occur, despite the best of care by the best of surgeons. As a general rule, a risk is a surgical complication that cannot be reduced or eliminated by skill, care, or technology. Skill refers to physical surgery and the use and control of instruments. Care refers to the diagnosis, planning, and follow-up of a patient, such as prescribing preoperative antibiotics. Technology refers to aids such as imaging, monitors, and testing. In contrast, when a complication results and there is a lack of skill, care, or failure to use technology, experts may testify that the complication is an injury caused by failure to meet the standard of care. The cases that follow are examples of complications with tips for avoidance of claims through practice management.

Extractions

Dental alveolar surgery typically comprises most of the procedures in an oral and maxillofacial surgery practice and is also the source of most of the claims of substandard care. Except for wrong site surgery, which is not a complication, most of these claims involve issues of whether the complication is a risk or the result of substandard care.

Nerve injuries, infections, and jaw fractures after dental alveolar surgery comprise many of the claims for malpractice, despite the fact that such

[Doctor's letterhead]

Date:_____   Fax No. _____

Dear Dr. _____: This fax will confirm our conversation of today wherein we discussed your

patient, _____, and his/her condition(s) of

_____

_____

and our proposed treatment of

_____

_____

[ ] with local anesthesia   [ ] with epinephrine   [ ] with [ ] without IV Sedation

scheduled for _____. In response, you recommended the

following:

_____

_____

_____

Thank you for your advice in this matter. Please immediately advise us before the next business day if this
letter is not accurate or if the patient's condition should significantly change before our scheduled
treatment/operation as noted above. Otherwise, we will proceed as noted and will assume the foregoing is
a correct statement of your advice.

_____

[Doctor's Name]

THE DOCUMENT BEING FAXED IS INTENDED ONLY FOR THE USE OF THE INDIVIDUAL OR ENTITY
TO WHICH IT IS ADDRESSED, AND IT MAY CONTAIN INFORMATION THAT IS PRIVILEGED, CONFIDENTIAL
AND EXEMPT FROM DISCLOSURE UNDER APPLICABLE LAW.

IF THE READER OF THIS MESSAGE IS NOT THE INTENDED RECIPIENT, YOU ARE HEREBY NOTIFIED
THAT ANY DISSEMINATION, DISTRIBUTION OR COPYING OF THIS COMMUNICATION IS STRICTLY
PROHIBITED. IF YOU HAVE RECEIVED THIS COMMUNICATION IN ERROR, PLEASE NOTIFY US IMMEDIATELY
BY TELEPHONE AND RETURN THE ORIGINAL MESSAGE TO THE ABOVE ADDRESS VIA THE UNITED STATES
POSTAL SERVICE.

Fig. 1. Confirmation letter for patient referral from another doctor.

complications can and do happen in the absence
of negligence.

Nerve injuries

Postextraction nerve injury cases associated with
extractions historically have involved both inferior
alveolar nerves (IAN) and lingual nerves as well as
claims of lack of informed consent and negligent
surgery. Before the widespread use of detailed
written consent forms in the late 1980s, the outcome of such cases turned on the credibility of
the witnesses (ie, the patient vs the surgeon) as to
what was or was not said. In cases where there
was evidence of a signed consent form, the

surgeon more often prevailed because the injury
was considered a risk of surgery. The result was
a significant drop in cases involving nerve injuries,
Currently, there are few claims involving injury to
the IAN. However, in the mid-1990s, claims involving lingual nerve damage began to increase. The
new tactic in these cases was to abandon the issue
of informed consent and focus instead on a claim of
negligent surgery. The plaintiffs retained surgeons
to testify that, because the lingual nerve is outside
the mandible, severance was the result of substandard surgery. Almost all the cases involved severe
or complete numbness rather than merely reduced
sensation.[22] The testimony was that, although mild

[Doctor's letterhead]

Date:_____   Fax No. _____

Dear Dr. _____ : This will introduce _____,

who is being referred to you for evaluation and/or treatment as you deem appropriate for his/her

condition(s) or potential of

_____

_____

The following will be sent [by mail] [with patient]

_____

This patient needs to be seen by _____[DATE]_____. If you have not been able to see or appoint the
patient by that date, please contact this office so that we may followup with the patient. Unless we hear to
the contrary, this letter will confirm that you have agreed to see, treat or evaluate the patient as you deem
necessary and appropriate.

_____

[Doctor's Name]

THE DOCUMENT BEING FAXED IS INTENDED ONLY FOR THE USE OF THE INDIVIDUAL OR ENTITY
TO WHICH IT IS ADDRESSED, AND IT MAY CONTAIN INFORMATION THAT IS PRIVILEGED, CONFIDENTIAL
AND EXEMPT FROM DISCLOSURE UNDER APPLICABLE LAW.

IF THE READER OF THIS MESSAGE IS NOT THE INTENDED RECIPIENT, YOU ARE HEREBY NOTIFIED
THAT ANY DISSEMINATION, DISTRIBUTION OR COPYING OF THIS COMMUNICATION IS STRICTLY
PROHIBITED. IF YOU HAVE RECEIVED THIS COMMUNICATION IN ERROR, PLEASE NOTIFY US IMMEDIATELY
BY TELEPHONE AND RETURN THE ORIGINAL MESSAGE TO THE ABOVE ADDRESS VIA THE UNITED STATES
POSTAL SERVICE.

Fig. 2. Introduction letter for patient referral to another doctor.

numbness could be caused by stretching, a needle, or bruising, significant or complete loss of sensation only could occur with partial or complete severance caused by either a drill bit or scalpel and, therefore, substandard care. In addition, many

cases of postoperative lingual anesthesia were followed by attempts at surgical repair and the operative findings were critical to the claim of severance. These factual scenarios resulted in some verdicts for patients.

Tips Many of the nonnegligent reasons for lingual nerve injury have not been well documented. Adequate documentation has been essential to defending and preventing such claims. At surgery, chart any unusual findings such as the absence of a lingual plate, a tenacious follicular sac, or even the finding of what appears to be nerve tissue on the crest of the bony socket. Photograph any such findings. The surgeon should call all patients at risk for nerve damage the evening of the surgery and chart their responses to questions regarding neurologic status, positive or negative. If negative, that could be evidence that any subsequent numbness was not the result of surgery but due to infection and/or scarring. If the response is positive, the patient should be scheduled for an

---

Box 1
Instructions for sending confirming letters by fax to health care providers

The fax machine should be set to:

• Print transmission data on an individual setting, not every 20 messages or so
• Each print should include a copy of the letter (either full-size or reduced), and at the top show all of the transmission data from the sender to the receiver
• The data should include date, time, number dialed, time taken to transmit, and result: either OK (showing number of pages sent), NG (for no good), or Error

examination using the neurologic examination form of the American Association of Oral and Maxillofacial Surgeons. Also consider photographing the site of the surgery and the areas of numbness. Based on accepted guidelines, consider recommendations or referral for early surgical repair and chart these discussions with the patient. In the event the clinical findings suggest that surgical repair may be beneficial and the patient declines the recommendation or referral, chart that informed refusal was obtained.

Jaw fractures

Patients are at risk for jaw fracture either during or after surgery. Most claims involve either failure to diagnose or late diagnosis with resulting injury claims of nerve damage or the need for surgical fracture fixation.

Tips Documentation is essential, beginning with the need for extraction. Clinical observations, such as periodontal pockets, pericornitis, pain, or swelling should be recorded in addition to radiographic findings. At discharge, the absence of any evidence of fracture should be noted for patients at risk. Patients should also be given detailed written postoperative instructions, the issuance of which should be recorded, along with any video presentations viewed by the patient. Subsequently, reports of unusually persistent pain or bite problems not associated with typical postoperative swelling should be noted and the patient scheduled for examination and, depending upon the clinical presentation, radiographs taken. Chart any report of patient activities at the onset of symptoms, such as eating hard foods, playing sports, or trauma. If any referrals are made and the patient declines, obtain written informed refusal.

Infections

Although not common, postoperative infections have been the source of some claims of substandard care, despite being a known risk and part of almost all written consent forms. The allegations typically are that the patient should have been given antibiotics either before or at discharge or that the surgeon ignored the patient's postoperative complaints and failed to diagnose and treat the infection in timely fashion, such that the patient suffered a more severe infection and/or required surgical intervention.[23] Sinus communications are at risk with extractions of upper molars and occasionally become the subject of claims due to late diagnosis.

Tips Document the clinical and radiographic findings that support the need for the extractions and whether preoperative or prophylactic antibiotics are indicated. If antibiotics are clinically

indicated and are offered and declined by the patient, chart informed refusal. At postoperative encounters, if a patient reports unusual persistent pain or swelling, consider an earlier postoperative examination. On examination, if upper teeth were involved, chart the lack of oroantral communications in patients at risk. Record subsequent return postoperative examination findings, including the patient's vital signs, even if normal, and any findings of lack of patient compliance with home care. It is particularly important to remain in close communication with such a patient to provide appropriate care and advice. Often claims originate because a patient cannot reach the surgeon or calls are not returned and the patient goes to another physician or emergency department, where more aggressive care is provided than would be indicated in the office of an experienced oral and maxillofacial surgeon.

Implants

One way to understand the claims issues with implant complications is to consider that they are really reverse extractions and, therefore, carry the same risks. The primary difference is that with extractions, the surgeon has no control over the location of the teeth and the surrounding structures. Whereas, with implants, the surgeon controls the placement of the implant relative to surrounding structures. Although the risks may be similar, the claims have been that the surgeon could or should have altered the location of the implant to reduce or eliminate the risk of complications. Most of the claims that have resulted in verdicts in favor of the plaintiffs have been associated with nerve injuries, particularly chronic severe pain alleged to be due to partial nerve damage rather than severance.[24]

Tips As with extractions, patient candidacy and the indications for implants should be charted. If adjunct procedures such as grafting or lifts are also indicated, and if a patient declines such recommendation, the informed refusal, including the risks of having no implant or the risks of an implant without a graft or sinus lift, should be documented.

Cone beam computed tomography (CBCT)

Claims have been made by experts for plaintiffs that the use of additional imaging such as cone beam computed tomography (CBCT) could have prevented such an injury. The experience of this author has been that imaging does not replace surgical judgment. Whether or not CBCT is a standard of care is subject to significant controversy, including the issue of excess or needless radiation exposure. For years, surgeons have successfully placed implants without the use of CBCT scans.

Computed tomography is not new technology and has been available to surgeons for many years. CBCT has reduced the size and costs of CT scanners, the amount of radiation, and the area of exposure. However, in this author's experience, most failures were either due to the patient's reaction to surgery (a risk) or poor judgment by the surgeon, rather than an imaging issue. CBCT is not a substitute for careful planning by the surgeon.

Tips The need for and the contribution of CBCT in implant placement should be evaluated by surgeons on a case-by-case basis. There is no rule of law that CBCT is the standard of care for all implant cases, particularly considering the additional costs and radiation exposure compared with panoramic films. However, if offered to a patient and declined, informed refusal should be obtained, charted, and signed by the patient. At surgery and postsurgery, surgeons are advised to follow the same protocols for documenting and evaluation as noted in the previous extraction comments. The primary difference is that implants can be removed and, in some cases, early removal can reduce or resolve neurologic symptoms. The surgeon is advised to document the clinical findings and the options given to the patient, such as implant removal and, if the patient declines, to document informed refusal. Clinical judgment will determine whether to remove the implant and let the area resolve or to immediately place a shorter implant. However, experts for plaintiffs have testified that, if the shorter implant would work, why was it not chosen in the first place to minimize the potential for injury. Therefore, document why a particular length of implant was chosen.

Sinus infections
Sinus infections are a risk of surgery with extractions and/or implant placement and/or sinus lifts. Most cases with good consent documentation do not result in claims. However, failure to diagnose and treat such infections in timely fashion can cause claims for malpractice.

Tips Close follow-up after surgery continues to be a good risk management tool, including the recording of the absence of problems or complaints at each encounter. The lack of documentation allows patients to claim that their complaints were ignored. If there are complaints suggestive of infection or sinus opening, a clinical examination should be performed and charted in detail, including the absence of any findings. Photos and vital signs are also recommended as evidence of the examination. Where indicated, consider imaging and/or referral to another specialist such as an otolaryngologist. If the patient declines or fails to follow the recommendation, obtain and chart informed refusal or the patient's lack of cooperation.

Grafts
Grafts have the same risks as extractions and implants, and it is recommended that the same protocols be followed for these surgeries as would be applied to extraction and implant complications.

Orthognathic procedures
With the drop in the number of orthognathic procedures being performed, the number of claims associated with such procedures also has dropped. However, such claims when they do occur, most often are associated with the lack of informed consent or surgical failure.

Tips Because of the complexity of the surgery, any issues and any medical consultations in the patient's health history that could affect healing should be noted. Detailed specific procedure consent forms should be used and well documented. Doing so will reduce most claims. In the event of a surgical failure, close follow-up and documentation, including the lack of symptoms and problems, should be noted. In the event of clinical findings of surgical failure, evaluation for correction or follow-up should be discussed with the patient and appropriate imaging considered where indicated. If the patient should decline imaging or further surgery, written informed refusal should be obtained. In any event, detailed operative reports are good risk management tools. Also, if any unusual findings are seen during surgery, such as unexpected anatomic aberrance, consider documentation by photograph before, during, and/or after surgery, in addition to imaging.

SUMMARY

Risks are complications that can and do occur, despite the best of care by the best of surgeons and in the absence of negligence. However, claims of negligent planning, surgery, and postoperative care have been made due primarily to poor documentation and lack of supporting evidence, such as images and photographs. Proactive documentation that includes charting the absence of contraindications to surgery and the presence or lack of unusual surgery findings, close follow-up care to include early encounters (calls or visits), making referrals, and obtaining informed refusal can significantly reduce claims of substandard care.

REFERENCES

1. Health Insurance Portability and Accountability Act, 45 C.F.R., 160 et seq., 1996.

2. Occupational Safety and Health Act, 29 U.S.C. 651 et seq., 1970.

3. Brown v Colm, 11 Cal.3d 639, 642B643, 1974.

4. Rowland v Christian, 69 Cal.2d 108, 111–112, 1968. California Civil Jury Instructions (CACI) 400, 500, 501 (2010).

5. Landeros v Flood, 17 Cal.3d 399, 410, 1976.

6. California Code of Civil Procedure Section 2034.210. 2010.

7. California Code of Civil Procedure Section 2034. 210(a). 2010.

8. California Code of Civil Procedure Section 2034. 210(b). 2010.

9. CDA Code of Ethics Section 10A. 2010.

10. California Evidence Code Section 721. 2010.

11. Available at: http://www.americanheart.org/presenter. jhtml?identifier=3047051. Accessed April 8, 2011.

12. Available at: http://www.asahq.org/For-Healthcare-Professionals/Standards-Guidelines-and-Statements.aspx. Accessed April 8, 2011.

13. Available at: http://www.aaomsstore.com/p-65-aaoms-parameters-of-care-clinical-practice-guidelines.aspx. Accessed April 8, 2011.

14. Available at: http://www.aaoms.org/docs/practice_mgmt/impairment_guidelines_2006.pdf. Accessed April 8, 2011.

15. Available at: http://www.justia.com/trials-litigation/docs/caci/400/405.html. Accessed April 8, 2011.

16. Beford v Zimerman, 262 Va. 81 (2001).

17. Available at: http://www.justia.com/trials-litigation/docs/caci/200/200.html. Accessed April 8, 2011.

18. Available at: http://law.onecle.com/california/business/2266.html. Accessed April 8, 2011.

19. Available at: http://www.justia.com/trials-litigation/docs/caci/500/532.html. Accessed April 8, 2011.

20. Available at: http://www.justia.com/trials-litigation/docs/caci/500/535.html. Accessed April 8, 2011.

21. Available at: http://www.courtinfo.ca.gov/rules/index.cfm?title=two&;linkid=rule2_306. Accessed April 8, 2011.

22. Available at: http://www.joms.org/article/S0278-2391(02)15642-4/abstract. Accessed April 8, 2011.

23. Available at: http://www.dentists-advantage.com/rskmgt/casestudy/getCase.jsp?id=349. Accessed April 8, 2011.

24. Available at: http://www.dentists-advantage.com/rskmgt/casestudy/getCase.jsp?id=296. Accessed April 8, 2011.

Index

Note: Page numbers of article titles are in **boldface** type.

Oral Maxillofacial Surg Clin N Am 23 (2011) 485–489
doi:10.1016/S1042-3699(11)00118-X
1042-3699/11/$ – see front matter © 2011 Elsevier Inc. All rights reserved.

Moving?

Make sure your subscription moves with you!

To notify us of your new address, find your **Clinics Account Number** (located on your mailing label above your name), and contact customer service at:

Email: journalscustomerservice-usa@elsevier.com

800-654-2452 (subscribers in the U.S. & Canada)
314-447-8871 (subscribers outside of the U.S. & Canada)

Fax number: 314-447-8029

Elsevier Health Sciences Division
Subscription Customer Service
3251 Riverport Lane
Maryland Heights, MO 63043

Moving?

Make sure your subscription moves with you!

To notify us of your new address, find your **Clinics Account Number** (located on your mailing label above your name), and contact customer service at:

Email: journalscustomerservice-usa@elsevier.com

800-654-2452 (subscribers in the U.S. & Canada)
314-447-8871 (subscribers outside of the U.S. & Canada)

Fax number: 314-447-8029

Elsevier Health Sciences Division
Subscription Customer Service
3251 Riverport Lane
Maryland Heights, MO 63043

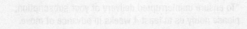

To ensure uninterrupted delivery of your subscription, please notify us at least 4 weeks in advance of move.

Printed and bound by CPI Group (UK) Ltd, Croydon, CR0 4YY

03/10/2024

01040010 0007